How to Hack your Vagus Nerve

Exercises to dramatically reduce Inflammation, Trauma and Anxiety with Vagal Stimulation

Katrina Power

TABLE OF CONTENTS

Introduction

A ll signals going up from the gut to the brain through the vagus nerve influences your possibility of satiation or having more cravings, as well as your mood and feelings of anxiety, and the initiation of your inflammatory stress reaction.

It's an extremely significant pathway, and vagus nerve initiation is associated with obesity, gastrointestinal illnesses, cardiovascular illnesses, disposition issues like depression, and a wide range of other incessant medical issues. Here's a look at why the vagus nerve is so significant, and how your eating routine can improve your wellbeing by influencing vagal nerve signals from the gut.

We are in possession of a wonderful system. A system that performs so many tasks simultaneously; its mind boggling when you take a moment to think about it. You are probably sitting somewhere, or you could be lying down. Your eyes travel across the page, grasping words and interpreting them instantly.

Your breathing, body temperature, heart rate, blinking, bowel movement, posture control, and thousands of other important decisions. Your heart doesn't simply stop beating and think to itself, *"Well, since this human is reading, I'll just take a 10-minute power nap."*

You never see that happen, unless a person has a heart condition that makes their heart function in abnormal ways.

Your nervous system plays a huge role in regulating your stress and happiness levels. For a long time now, the commonly held belief has been that the autonomic nervous system largely functions in two states: relaxation and stress. This theory is so widespread that doctors and psychologists to this day prescribe treatments for stress, anxiety, and depression based on it.

Most of you might ponder to yourself, what is a vagus nerve? How important is it to the body? And how is it connected to taking care of the body, helping it heal and maintain optimal health?

In this book we will learn about the vagus nerve in detail. For now, understand that this nerve plays a vital role in our body such as contributing to our immune system and helping us manage our mental health. Some of its other functions include releasing testosterone and bile, regulating blood glucose and blood pressure, assisting with saliva secretion, and promoting healthy kidney function.

Chapter 1: Introduction to the Autonomic Nervous System

The Autonomic Nervous System

T he autonomic nervous system is a part of the nervous system that controls the bodily functions that we are not consciously aware of or control ourselves. In order for us to understand the autonomic nervous system, we need to know that the nervous system is made up of two opposing systems that are constantly sending information back and forth the brain and back to the organs.

The sympathetic side of the autonomic nervous system is mostly in control of your energy levels, alertness during the course of the day, your blood pressure, breathing, and heart rate.

This part of the system prepares us to act when it is needed and greatly affects hormones that give you your fight or flight reactions, namely adrenaline and cortisol levels. The parasympathetic side of the nervous system, which contains most of the vagus nerve's functions and which the vagus nerve is greatly a part of, is there to decrease alertness, help with calming effects on the body, lower your heart rate and blood pressure, as well as aid your body with relaxation in stressful moments and help with digestion. Because the vagus nerve is a large part of the parasympathetic system, it also plays a role in helping with urination and defecation as well as sparking sexual arousal!

You can picture these two systems working together much like the accelerator and the brake in a car.

The sympathetic nervous system would be your accelerator and it gets us up and going with all the energy in the world, and then when it comes time to calm down and relax, the parasympathetic nervous system will be your decelerator and will therefore reduce the speed at which we are going, and will then use certain neurotransmitters such as acetylcholine in order to lower your blood pressure and heart rate and cause the organs of the body to slow down their processes, too.

What Is the Autonomic Nervous System?

Certainly, you are familiar with the term 'nervous system.' It is a complex part of the body that is responsible for automatically coordinating the body's actions and sensory information by sending signals from one part of the body to another. It performs this task through a special type of cell called a neuron or a nerve cell.

The nervous system consists of two main parts: the central nervous system (CNS) and the peripheral nervous system (PNS). The CNS is made up of the brain and spinal cord, the importance of which is obvious. The brain controls all body functions including movement, awareness, thought, speech, memory, and much more. The spinal cord is linked to a portion of the brain called the brainstem where it sends messages from the brain to the peripheral nerves and vice versa, and it also plays a very vital role in body positioning.

The peripheral nervous system can be said to oversee all activities which take place in the body apart from the brain and spinal cord, or the CNS. Its primary role is to ensure that the various body parts are communicating well and working in harmony. When communication is at its peak, we will be able to react appropriately to the various stimuli we sense from the environment.

You are probably asking yourself where the autonomic nervous system fits into all of this.

Relax... stay with me. You will soon find out.

The peripheral nervous system is further divided into two parts: the somatic nervous system and the autonomic nervous system (ANS).

Aha... Now we're talking...

The word 'somatic' is derived from the Greek word 'soma' which means 'body.' This implies that the somatic nervous system is responsible for sending and receiving motor and sensory information either to or from the CNS. It is also a major player in voluntary movement. To this effect, this system consists of two major types of neurons, sensory and motor neurons, which carry information from the body to the brain and spinal cord, and from the brain and spinal cord to the body, respectively. It is their actions that result in a response to physical stimuli.

Finally, there is the autonomic nervous system. The ANS is otherwise called the 'Vegetative Nervous System.' It is a part of the peripheral nervous system that directly controls the function of internal organs such as glands, blood vessels, genitals, lungs, heart, smooth muscles, *etc.* This system carries out activities in the body unconsciously or without thought, such as respiration, heart rate, urination, digestion, and sexual arousal, for example. It is also in charge of the fight-flight-freeze response. This theory was first discovered by the intellectual Walter Cannon.

The ANS is controlled by the hypothalamus in the brain. This means that the hypothalamus controls the autonomic or automatic functions such as breathing, and the heartbeat and reflexes such as sneezing, vomiting and coughing. These functions are still subdivided into different areas and are linked to the subsystems of the ANS. The hypothalamus, which is located just a bit above the brain stem, integrates these autonomic functions. This system is one of the most important systems in the human body, as any disorder of this system may be progressive or irreversible and can affect the entire body.

Now the ANS is divided into three systems: the sympathetic nervous system, the parasympathetic nervous system and the enteric nervous system, but the major systems are the first two. The enteric nervous system hasn't yet been globally recognized as part of the ANS, and some textbooks do not even include it. Therefore, we will start with the first two.

What is the Sympathetic Nervous System?

Think about your past or current fears. Whether we admit it or not, most of us have fears, whether mild or extreme.

The way you respond to fear is known as the fight-flight-freeze response (or the acute stress response). This response is controlled and managed by the sympathetic nervous system. It is usually active at a low level to regulate homeostasis, which is the equilibrium and harmony in the body.

Interesting, isn't it? So how does it work?

Sympathetic nerves begin in the central nervous system in the sections of the spine known as the thoracic spine and the lumbar spine. It is sometimes referred to as the thoracolumbar outflow because the axons or ends of these cells exit the spine here, and communicate or synapse with either sympathetic ganglion cells (which connect to and regulate various organs including the heart) or the specialized cells in the kidneys and the adrenal glands (which sit on top of the kidneys).

Sympathetic neurons emit neurotransmitters or chemicals called epinephrine and norepinephrine (also known as adrenaline and noradrenaline). Adrenaline, as we know, jumpstarts the body into action, with effects such as increasing the heart rate, diverting the blood flow from the organs toward the skeletal muscles, dilating the pupils and increasing sweating, for example.

Sympathetic nerves that connect to the kidneys release a chemical called dopamine. Dopamine can be turned into norepinephrine (noradrenaline) in the adrenal glands if the body signals for it. Sympathetic nerves that connect to the chromaffin cells in the adrenal glands produce substantial amounts of epinephrine (adrenaline) from norepinephrine. Both epinephrine and norepinephrine result in responses that ready the body for action under stress.

Why is this system known as the 'sympathetic' nervous system, of all things? History has it that this name stems from the idea of sympathy. Sympathy is the perception of someone's or something's distress and reacting accordingly, so it was thought of in the sense of having a connection between parts or people. It was first used medically by Claudius Galenus (otherwise known as Galen of Pergamon). But in the 18th century, it was used specifically for nerves by French anatomist, Jacob B. Winslow.

Now we will address the second part of the autonomic nervous system.

The Parasympathetic Nervous System

The autonomic nervous system regulates the unconscious actions of the body, and the Parasympathetic Nervous System (PSNS) controls the unconscious activities that take place when the body is at rest, often after eating. These activities include salivation, lacrimation (tear flow), sexual arousal, digestion, urination, defecation, *etc.* and they are often known as the 'feed and breed' or 'rest and digest' activities. The function of the PSNS complements that of the sympathetic nervous system, which regulates fight-flight-freeze responses.

Parasympathetic nerves have a craniosacral outflow (they exit the CNS from the brain stem or from the sacral region of the spine), compared to the sympathetic system that has a thoracolumbar outflow.

The nerves in this system are autonomic, and their supply primarily stems from these three sources: the cranial nerves, the vagus nerve and the pelvic splanchnic nerves.

Parasympathetic nerves (a special type of cranial nerve) stem from a particular nuclei (groups of nerve cells in the CNS) and form a synapse at any of the four parasympathetic ganglia (groups of nerve cells outside the CNS or in the PNS). It is from there that these nerves reach their target tissues through trigeminal nerves (nerves that are responsible for motor and sensory functions). Another type of cranial nerve is called the oculomotor nerve, which regulates most of the eye-related parasympathetic functions.

The vagus nerve originates in the lower half of the brain stem which is connected to the spinal cord (known as the brain stem medulla). The term 'vagus nerve' originates from the Latin word 'vagus' which means 'wandering.' This is appropriate considering that this nerve controls a lot of target tissues. However, the vagus nerve is quite unusual because it doesn't follow the trigeminal nerve path to get to its destination (the target tissues). Also, this nerve is very difficult to trace because it is virtually everywhere in the thorax and abdomen. As such, several parasympathetic nerves leave the vagus nerve as they enter the thorax, such as the laryngeal and cardiac nerves. The organs affected by the parasympathetic nerves in the abdomen include the pancreas, kidney and gall bladder among others.

The pelvic splanchnic nerves exit the spine through the sacral region. They contribute immensely to the supply of nerves to the genital and pelvic organs. They regulate urinary excretion, the sensation of pain, and sexual functions like penis erection.

Remember when it was stated that the parasympathetic nervous system has a **craniosacral** outflow? The pelvic splanchnic nerves are an important **sacral** component of the PSNS. It is in the same location as the sacral splanchnic nerves that emerge from the sympathetic trunk in the SNS.

Parasympathetic nerves produce the neurotransmitter acetylcholine, which is received by the target organs which respond by stimulating parasympathetic activities.

Relationship between the Sympathetic and Parasympathetic Nervous Systems

The interesting thing about the sympathetic and parasympathetic components of the autonomic nervous system is that they work opposite each other. First, the SNS controls actions that require a quick and immediate response, while the PSNS controls slower or delayed activities. Furthermore, the SNS speeds up the body processes, for example, increasing the heart rate when faced with imminent danger. The PSNS on the other hand calms the body, for example reducing the heart rate.

Muscles stimulated by the SNS contract, while those stimulated by the PSNS relax. The SNS releases adrenaline, while the PSNS has no connection with the adrenal gland. The same goes for glycogen conversion; the SNS transforms glycogen into glucose for muscle energy. The bronchial tubes constrict when influenced by the PSNS but dilate under the influence of the SNS. There is an increase in urinary output when the PSNS is active, while the opposite happens with the SNS activity. The neurons in the PSNS are cholinergic (produce and receive acetylcholine), while in the SNS neurons are adrenergic (produce and receive norepinephrine/epinephrine).

The Enteric Nervous System (ENS)

Otherwise known as the intrinsic nervous system, the ENS is one of the systems in the ANS. Its system of neurons in the lining of the gastrointestinal tract regulate the activities of the GI tract from the esophagus, all the way down to the anus. One powerful thing about this system is that it can work without the sympathetic and parasympathetic systems, but may be affected by them. The ENS, also more trendily known as the gut, is sometimes referred to as the second brain.

This system operates without the brain and the spinal cord but needs the supply of nerves from the autonomic nervous system through the prevertebral ganglia and vagus nerve. However, research has shown that the enteric nervous system can function even with a severed vagus nerve. The neurons from this system not only secrete enzymes from the gastrointestinal tract but also regulate motor functions.

The ENS contains over 500 million neurons. There are over 100 million neurons in the spinal cord alone. These neurons interact via neurotransmitters that are almost the same as those used in the CNS, and they include dopamine, serotonin and acetylcholine.

The Function of the Autonomic Nervous System in the Body

Recall that the autonomic nervous system is a division of the peripheral nervous system, which is a division of the nervous system as a whole. The ANS is responsible for regulating functions that are carried out without conscious effort. Then it was also stated that the ANS has two divisions, the sympathetic nervous system (SNS) and the parasympathetic nervous system (PSNS).

It would therefore be fitting to say that the functions of the ANS are the functions of the individual divisions. The SNS takes care of the fight-or-flight responses. The PSNS takes care of the actions the body undertakes at rest, especially after eating. The ENS takes care of the activities of the gastrointestinal tract.

Functions of the Sympathetic Nervous System

1. It regulates homeostasis.

This function does not just apply to human beings but to all living organisms. The fibers in this system supply nerves to the tissues of almost every organ in the body. This process regulates diverse functions like blood flow, urinary control, pupil dilation and constriction, body temperature, blood sugar levels, pH, *etc.*

2. It regulates the fight-or-flight response, sometimes called fight-flight-freeze response or the sympathoadrenal response (derived from the words 'sympathetic' and 'adrenal medulla').

This is one of the most important functions of the SNS. It controls the hormonal and neuronal stress response in a way that the preganglionic fibers in the system activate the release of epinephrine (adrenaline) in great quantities, acting directly on the cardiovascular system. When activated, the SNS or fight-or-flight response:

- Constricts blood vessels, especially those in the kidney and skin. This happens when the adrenergic receptors are activated by norepinephrine that is released by postganglionic neurons. This also causes a redirection of blood flow from the skin and gastrointestinal tract.

- Boosts blood flow to the lungs and skeletal muscles.

- Allows the coronary vessels of the heart to widen or relax, especially the ones in large arteries, large veins and smaller arterioles.

- Prevents peristalsis, thereby preventing digestion.

3. It gets the body ready for action, especially in life-threatening situations.

For instance, the SNS prepares your body in the morning before you wake up by increasing its outflow spontaneously.

4. It relaxes the ciliary muscles.

These are found in the eye and are linked to the lens and dilates the pupils, thereby allowing more light to penetrate the eye.

5. It dilates the bronchioles of the lungs by spreading epinephrine continuously, thereby improving the oxygen exchange.

6. It increases the heart rate.

The contribution of both the sympathetic and parasympathetic nervous systems to the sinoatrial node regulates the heart rate. Note that the heart rate is different from the heart rhythm. Heart rate is the number of times the heart beats per second, while the heart rhythm is the pattern in which the heart beats. When the heart rate is increased, the blood flow to the heart and active skeletal muscles is improved.

7. It stimulates sweat excretion in the sweat glands.

8. It prevents tumescence or swelling.

Penis tumescence is commonly known as penis erection, which entails blood filling the penis in preparation for sexual activity. When faced with life-threatening situations, the SNS prevents this from occurring.

9. It constricts all the intestinal and urinary sphincters.

10. It activates orgasm.

Functions of the Parasympathetic Nervous System

Recall that the parasympathetic nervous system functions directly opposite to the sympathetic nervous system. The PSNS:

1. It aids sexual activity.

2. The nerves in this system help to erect the genital tissues through the pelvic splanchnic nerves. When a man is about to ejaculate, the sympathetic system causes the internal pelvic sphincter to close and the urethral muscle to undergo peristalsis. Likewise, the parasympathetic system causes peristalsis to occur in the urethral muscle, and the bulbospongiosus muscles are contracted by the pudendal nerve to violently discharge the semen. The penis becomes flaccid again afterwards.

3. Increases blood flow by relaxing or widening blood vessels that are linked to the gastrointestinal tract.

4. Enhances near vision by contracting the pupil and constricting the ciliary muscles in the eye. This is

the exact opposite of what the SNS does, which is enhancing far vision.

5. Improves absorption of nutrients by enhancing the secretion of saliva and the rate of peristalsis.

6. Reduces the diameter of the bronchioles when the body needs less oxygen.

7. Lowers the heart rate by producing acetylcholine, contrary to the sympathetic nervous system which increases heart rate by producing epinephrine and norepinephrine (or adrenaline and noradrenaline).

Functions of the Enteric Nervous System

The ENS (also known as the second brain) has its own unique function since it is the nervous system that coordinates the processes of the gastrointestinal system. The ENS:

1. Acts as a neuron integrating unit. This system is called the second brain primarily because it can exist on its own. It interacts with the CNS through the pre-vertebral ganglia and the vagus nerve, but it can still function autonomously when the vagus nerve is severed.

2. Because this system is made up of several kinds of neurons (neurons that both send and receive signals), it can stand in for the CNS input as an integrating unit. These neurons act on chemical and mechanical conditions.

3. It controls GI tract secretions. Gastrointestinal enzymes are controlled by cholinergic neurons that are located on the walls of the digestive tract.

Importance of the Vagus Nerve

The vagus nerve is in charge of a vast range of key bodily functions, constantly communicating sensory and motor impulses to each and every organ of the body. Recent studies have even revealed that this 'wanderer' may be the missing link in the treatment of chronic inflammation. Some even dare to claim that it could be the beginning of the discovery of treatment for many serious illnesses that are currently considered incurable. The following are a few of the many fascinating facts about this incredible nerve bundle that scientists are only beginning to discover.

It Helps Form Memories

Psychologists from the University of Virginia conducted a study that concluded how stimulating the vagus nerve results in the release of norepinephrine into the amygdala. The vagus nerve carries messages to and from the brain, and this release of the said neurotransmitter helps strengthen the storage of memory in the brain's limbic regions. This region of the brain regulates arousal, as well as memory and feeling responses influenced by the emotional stimuli.

It Aids in Breathing

One of the main things that the vagus nerve does is elicit the neurotransmitter acetylcholine, which in turn tells the lungs to breathe. This is the reason that Botox is considered dangerous, since it interrupts the production of acetylcholine. It's a good thing, however, that the vagus nerve can also be stimulated to assist one's breathing. There are several vagal maneuvers that have been found to help stimulate the vagus nerve and improve breathing, which in turn reduces not only stress and anxiety, but anger, as well. These maneuvers can also reduce inflammation by activating the relaxation response of the parasympathetic nervous system.

It Reduces Inflammation

While inflammation is a normal part of the body's healing process, an overabundance of it has been linked to a number of diseases and medical conditions. What's amazing about the vagus nerve is that it has an anti-inflammatory effect. Acetylcholine and noradrenaline, the two major autonomic neurotransmitters, are highly involved in the immune regulation, particularly in relation to the inflammation through a variety of molecular pathways. According to recent studies, there is a connection between the immune system and the nervous system. These studies found out that the 'inflammatory reflex' is dependent upon the signals produced by the vagus nerve. This reflex is enabled by a neural circuit responsible for the regulation of the immune response to invasion and injury.

It Aids the Heart Function

The vagus nerve is intimately involved with the heart as most people know. It's the one responsible for regulating the heart by sending electrical impulses to the specialized muscle tissues acting as natural pacemakers. These specialized muscle tissues are located in the right atrium, where the acetylcholine released by the vagus nerve controls the pulse. Doctors can determine the heart rate variability of an individual or HRV, simply by measuring the time between individual heart beats and then plotting the results on a chart. With the data collected via this process, doctors can gain insight on the health of a person's heart, as well as their vagus nerve.

It Initiates Relaxation

Every time the body's sympathetic nervous system turns on the fight or flight response and pours adrenaline and the stress hormone cortisol into your brain and the rest of your body, it's the vagus nerve that tells your body to relax. It does this by releasing acetylcholine. Since the vagus nerve extends throughout the body and into many organs, it can easily send instructions to those parts like a fiber-optic cable would do. It then releases enzymes and proteins, such as oxytocin, vasopressin, and prolactin, all of which are designed to help the body calm down when stressed. In relation to this, individuals who have a stronger vagus response have a higher chance to recover more quickly after getting ill, injured, or after experiencing severe stress.

It Passes Information between the Brain and the Gut

The fact that people experience 'butterflies in the stomach' is proof of how strongly the brain is connected to the gut. Recent studies have discovered how the brain affects the gut health and vice versa, and this connection between the two is referred to as the gut-brain axis. The brain and the central nervous system is filled with neurons that tell the rest of the body how to behave.

Chapter 2: The Polyvagal Theory

T he polyvagal theory fully explains the way our autonomous nervous system (ANS) really works. You will recall that the ANS was previously explained via the two-state model, which were named stress and relaxation. In biological circles, these were named sympathetic and parasympathetic. While not totally invalid, there are a lot of holes in this view of what is a very complex system.

The two-state theory considered the vagus nerve as being just one big nerve, and this is clearly incorrect. Such conclusions were brought about from a failure to view the problem from different angles, thanks to adhering to the age old theories. The polyvagal theory changes all of that and helps us understand not only the nature of depression and anxiety better, but also their treatments.

The vagus nerve is at the center of the polyvagal theory and we've looked at it in great detail this far. Let's now take a step back and consider the theory as a whole.

Thermostats

The best way to think of these three levels of the ANS is to liken them to a thermostat. The nerves in your body monitor your sensory responses and initiate the appropriate reaction. A good example of this is our physical reactions to our environment. When we feel cold, our body begins shivering. The muscle shivers produce additional heat. We can then place ourselves close to a source of heat or simply wear more layers of clothing to protect ourselves better.

The responses of our ANS can be hybrid as well. Hybrid here refers to a combination of two layers. Friendly competition is an example of a hybrid between the ventral circuit and the sympathetic nervous system. The result is a simulation of a fight or flight state but has none of the bad side effects. An expression of physical intimacy is a hybrid between the dorsal and ventral state as explained previously.

Together with the hybrid states, we have five states that the ANS operates in, which is a far more flexible model of behavioral response as compared to the old relaxation versus stress model. Let's examine the ins and outs of the

ANS a bit more, and see how the cranial nerves play a role in all of this.

Neural Pathways

The first neural pathway, that is the ventral system, expresses itself through CN X (the vagus nerve) along with four other nerves, namely CN V, VII, IX and XI. This circuit promotes a soothing and relaxed feeling, which makes us socially amiable and open. In addition to this, emotions such as joy, positivity, and love are associated with the ventral branch of the vagus nerve.

Behaviorally, it expresses itself through shared time and activities with friends, family, and loved ones. In evolutionary terms, cooperation increased our chances of survival and this is why social activity brings us a lot of positive emotions. Even introverts and loners (people who like being alone) need a basic level of social connection since this is hardwired into all of us, even if the degree to which we need this is different (Oschman, 2016). Talking, walking, singing, dancing together and so on are just expressions of this need, as is making the decision to raise and nurture children.

The next neural pathway is the sympathetic nervous system as you know. This can also be referred to as the spinal sympathetic chain since most of the information with regards to this state is passed to the relevant organs via spinal nerves. This is when we beat ourselves up for movement, whether it be towards fighting or fleeing. Either way, survival is the ultimate aim here.

You can also think of this state resulting from your body being mobilized by fear. Emotions such as fear, anger, rage, and so on are associated with this neural pathway. When the sympathetic nervous system proves unequal to the task of dealing with the challenges we face, the dorsal system kicks in, and this is the third neural pathway.

When faced with imminent destruction, our brain decides to immobilize us and chooses to conserve whatever energy is left. As I highlighted earlier, immobilization can be an effective survival tactic in nature when the odds are highly against a creature. In human beings the emotions of helplessness, apathy, and hopelessness are associated with this pathway. Physically speaking, your blood pressure drops, your muscles become loose and bodily functions realign themselves as described earlier. You might even faint or go into shock.

The ultimate aim of the nervous system with all of these circuits is to maintain what is called homeostasis.

Homeostasis refers to a state of dynamic equilibrium between a living organism and its environment. In other words, your reaction to your environment needs to be appropriate. Laughing at danger is a singularly un-homeostasis like behavior.

Neuroception

Neuroception was the term coined by Stephen Porges to describe the process by which neural circuits distinguish between safe and unsafe situations. The thing with neuroception is that it occurs outside of our conscious awareness (Oschman, 2016). In fact, it takes place in the deeply primitive portion of our brain and reacts automatically. Experiences of having a sixth sense and so on are examples of neuroception.

This doesn't mean our conscious mind doesn't pick up information. The decision-making process is a complex interplay between the conscious and the subconscious portions of our brain. You can think of neuroception as being the processing of information that our conscious mind doesn't pick up. As such, it works a lot faster than the conscious perception. How many times have you walked into a situation and just known something was wrong? Alternatively, how often have you started doing something and everything just felt right? This is neuroception in action.

As you can see, there is plenty of room for things to go wrong as well. If your neuroception is warped, then you'll end up categorizing a perfectly normal situation as being abnormal and everything you perceive will be colored by this initial thought. This is referred to as priming in psychological circles (Oschman, 2016). Priming can be thought of as defining the frame your mind is in. If you witness an act of kindness prior to walking into a tough negotiation, you're more likely to view the other side as being amicable to a win/win situation.

Priming explains why the social media and the news tend to make us feel miserable, since all we see is hatred and stories of doom. When primed to believe the worst, you end up screening those very things into your life. Faulty neuroception can occur for a variety of reasons, ranging from deep seated trauma to short term priming.

You might be hungry and hence, are cranky. Therefore, you are less likely to put up with randomness in your activities. An example of deep-seated trauma might be the way people react to dogs. There is evidence that human beings have effectively bred every single hostile fiber out of dogs to the point where dogs these days are compelled to be friendly towards everything except predators (Oschman, 2016).

Despite this, some people are scared of dogs, thanks to their childhood trauma. If a person was attacked by a dog as a child, they're likely to always believe that a charging dog wants to attack them. This is irrespective of whether the charging dog wants to play or attack. Neuroception ensures a faulty diagnosis of the situation. Generally speaking, neuroception is extremely open to manipulation.

Psychological triggers exist everywhere, and some deep-seated trigger might prejudice us in a given situation. We might be deeply in love with someone and we might not be able to see their flaws. We can literally be blinded by love, in other words. Chemical substances and medication can interfere with our neuroception as well. Antidepressants inhibit hormones and affect our perception of events as we've already seen.

It isn't just emotional matters that neuroception affects. Homeostatic perception is also affected. For example, some types of medication affect the brain's ability to detect cold. In such circumstances, you will not shiver,

and your body will not react to the cold until you suffer
from hypothermia and die.

Trauma and Neuroception

Trauma plays an important role in the way we perceive
things. Those who suffer from conditions such as PTSD,
have a tough time classifying things as being non-
threatening, and face huge challenges in managing their
triggers. One of the reasons trauma is particularly
challenging is due to the manner in which the brain
learns and absorbs information.

The brain is a series of cells called neurons which are
interconnected with one another to form what is called a
neural network (Oschman, 2016). These networks
together form a body of information. When sensory input
is received, the connections fire up and a perception is
formed. In turn the appropriate ANS pathway is activated
to maintain homeostasis with the perceived environment.

The biggest weak link in all of this is neuroception. This is
the filter through which we view the world and it is
absurdly easy to manipulate as we've seen. Deeply
emotional experiences, positive or negative, can color
neuroception to the point where we turn facts on their
head and become blind to everything else.

A good example of this is the standard of political debate. Political debate has never been of a high standard, contrary to popular perception. One reason for this is the need for people to cling onto their perception (neuroception) no matter what. Social media is one giant affirmation machine which only shows us the things we like to see. As a result, our biases build and the existing neural networks become stronger.

The brain is predisposed to minimizing the effort it must take to arrive at a decision. This is the goal of learning, after all. When you sit down to drive your car, you don't want your brain to go over the entire learning process all over again. You'd never reach anywhere if this happened. While this learning and reduction of effort is very helpful when it comes to driving, brushing your teeth, cooking your food and so on, it is actively harmful when it comes to neuroception which is colored by trauma.

Your brain simply reacts the way it always has and when you try to challenge this existing behavior, it simply rebels. After all, what is the need to do things differently? Remember that learning new things requires effort and this is also why we learn far less as we grow older when compared to children. We simply don't wish to make the effort.

It's a lot easier to cling onto what we already know and keep hammering it, even if we know it's wrong or not based on fact, since the alternative is just too much work. So what is the point of all this discussion? Well, for one thing, changing habits and beliefs requires you to apply an equal and opposite force.

In other words, you need to perform new behaviors and new mindsets with a high degree of positive emotion (why would you want to adopt a negative emotion on purpose after all?) and then repeat the action over and over. This is how learning takes place. Using the exercises, I will highlight a few chapters from now that can make the learning process easier for you, since you'll be priming yourself for adopting new ways of thinking and improving your life.

All in all, polyvagal theory will help you become more aware of which mental state you're in. This awareness alone is powerful enough to snap you out of your current mind and push you into another state. I'm not saying you should expect miracles. However, is change possible? It absolutely is!

Chapter 3: Cranial Nerves; Function and Disorders

Your vagus nerve is a cranial nerve, one of the twelve pairs of nerve sets that are a direct line of communication from the body to the brain. Aside from this handful of nerve pairs, the rest of your body is only able to connect to the brain through the spine. This is why a severance of the spine can lead to paralysis; all of that feedback to your body is through the spinal column and the nerves that make up the spinal cord, and when that gets damaged, you run into a problem of no longer having a means of communication from the brain to the body.

The cranial nerves, however, do not require this. They bypass the spinal cord altogether and run throughout the body in order to serve their functions. For the most part, these nerves are tied to senses; they connect the various sensory organs to the brain and allow you to process information such as sight, smell, taste, and other sensory stimuli. This refers to their sensory functions; they are afferent and bring the information straight to the brain. However, cranial nerves also allow for the creation of motor functions. These allow for movement to occur within the areas that are sensing something. You may be able to move your eyes to track something that is moving, for example, or move your tongue.

The vagus nerve is just one of these pairs of nerves; it is commonly referred to as the 10th cranial nerve, and it is quite important. While all of your cranial nerves are important to varying degrees, what is important to note is that the vagus nerve is one of the more complex ones. It is particularly important due to the fact that it is a lifeline of communication between the body and the brain. Without this connection and communication, you run the risk of not being able to properly function your body. We will primarily be focusing on this particular nerve.

Cranial Nerves

The parasympathetic nervous system is the soothing balm that your body needs. When you're in this state, your brain is relaxed and you're able to access more of your faculties. You become more social automatically, and all the systems that were sidelined by the body under sympathetic conditions are reactivated and you begin to function normally, or as normally as a human being ought to.

Just as how our perception defines the activation of the sympathetic nervous system, the parasympathetic nervous system's activation depends on how we perceive the stimuli we receive. The system itself consists of 12 cranial nerves. Cranial refers to the fact that the nerves originate in the brain and innervate (or are present in) various organs throughout the body. Each of these nerves control a different function (Schulmann, 2019).

Olfactory Nerve (CN I)

This nerve is responsible for your sense of smell and it carries the information of a particular smell to your brain. Your brain then matches it to the existing memories and relays appropriate information throughout your body.

Optic Nerve (CN 11)

As the name suggests, this nerve is all about your sense of sight. What you see is communicated to the brain and the brain decides how it would like to perceive it.

Oculomotor Nerve (CN III)

This nerve innervates and provides motor function to the muscles around your eyes as well as your pupil's response to light. It doesn't control all of the muscles around your eyes but four of the six that are present.

Trochlear Nerve (CN IV)

This controls the muscle that is responsible for the downward, inward, and outward eye movement.

Trigeminal Nerve (CN V)

This is the second largest of all the cranial nerves and has both sensory and motor functions. As such, it has three distinct sections all of which innervate different portions of your face and are responsible for different functions ranging from your forehead, ears, nose, lips, and cheeks.

Abducens Nerve (CN VI)

This controls the lateral rectus muscle which is responsible for the eye movement towards the outside.

Facial Nerve (CV VII)

CN VII innervates your face and is responsible for a large number of sensory and motor functions. Despite its name, it also has functions with regards to your sense of taste as well as your tear ducts and glands.

Vestibulocochlear Nerve (CN VIII)

This mouthful of a nerve controls a lot of functions that has to do with your sense of hearing and balance. It has two branches, one of which innervates the inner ear and the other which tracks the movement of your head.

Glossopharyngeal Nerve (CN IX)

This has motor and sensory functions that has to do with the back of your throat, tongue, and your sinuses. It controls the movement of those muscles as well as relays information about them to your brain.

Vagus Nerve (CN X)

This is the hero of this book, and you'll learn all about it shortly.

Accessory Nerve (CN XI)

This controls the muscles in your neck and allows you to rotate and flex the muscles in that part of your body.

Hypoglossal Nerve (CN XII)

This controls the movement of your jaw and the muscles in your tongue.

Chapter 4: Vagus Nerve

What is the Vagus Nerve?

Y our vagus nerve is a pair of nerves that travel from the brain and down into the torso. It is the largest of the cranial nerves, traveling to interact with the majority of your internal organs. The vagus nerve is responsible for your parasympathetic nervous system, in particular, making it a major part of the autonomic system within your body. We will be discussing what the autonomic nervous system is in more detail in the next chapter, but for now, think of it as being specifically related to the automatic functions of the body. Your autonomic nervous system keeps your body functioning properly and makes sure that everything that you do is particularly tailored, to ensure that you can survive in the world around you.

This primarily happens through emotions. Your vagus nerve, in particular, can cause you to calm down through the activation of the parasympathetic nervous system. This tells the body to stop and calm down somewhat in order to ensure that you are able to stop and digest rather than exist in a fight or flight mode.

Your vagus nerve will begin at the back of your neck, connected to the brain at the brainstem. It leaves the skull without ever entering the spinal column, which makes it unique compared to the rest of the nerves in your body. It then travels throughout the neck and into the intrapleural area. It then connects to the heart and lungs to regulate and sense them, as well as to the ear. You then have your nerve travel into the epiglottis and the pharynx, as it travels down into the neck and vocal folds. It is only at that point that it then ventures elsewhere throughout the body.

At this point, it wanders further, going down to the guts. It connects to the smooth muscles within the gastrointestinal and respiratory tracts in order to control them. This connection is what allows for the gut-brain axis; the communication between your gut and your brain, as the name implies.

All of this happens with many different functions. The nerve needs to do all sorts of different functionalities in order to ensure that you are actually able to run your body properly. Without the vagus nerve, or when the vagus nerve is faulty in some way, you start to run into all sorts of problems, ranging from mental health issues, such as anxiety or depression, or even physical problems related to the immune system. When you cannot regulate out your vagus nerve, you cannot ensure that your body works well.

We have been watching the vagus nerve closely in modern science. It has been found that you can stimulate the vagus nerve when it does not work properly, and in doing so, you ensure that you are actually able to keep it functioning. You effectively shock it into working to allow for the regulation of symptoms related to inflammatory diseases, treatment-resistant depression, and many others as well. It has even been found to help manage epilepsy. We will be going into detail about this later, but for now, keep in mind that you can actually individually stimulate the vagus nerve in order to tap into its power.

Anatomy of the Vagus Nerve

The vagus nerve can primarily be divided into two different portions in order to understand it: the dorsal vagal complex and the ventral vagal complex. We will be looking at how this nerve goes through the body and allows for the visceral experiences of the body. They are primarily responsible for stress responses within mammals. There are parts that are more primitive that will lead you to freeze, such as playing dead when you are being pursued by something. There are other functions that are more evolved and more responsible for social settings. We will be looking at it all when considering the ways in which this nerve functions. In looking at these two branches of the vagus nerve, you can begin to understand how the body responds to stress and why you do what you do. Usually, the primitive systems are less prioritized than the others; they are there to be activated as a sort of last-ditch effort to keep you alive. After all, they are primitive for a reason; you have evolved new methods that are supposed to be better for you in general.

Dorsal Vagal Complex

The dorsal branch begins at the dorsal motor nucleus and is typically recognized to be the older of the two branches. It is primarily unmyelinated, referring to the fact that it does not have a myelin sheath in the way that most of your neurons do. This myelination is what allows for nerves to fire at a quicker rate than they otherwise would. Most vertebrates have this particular nerve, regardless if they are mammals or reptiles; it allows for the basic freeze response that you would see when you scare an animal. Frogs and lizards, when threatened, typically freeze. This allows for a conservation of the energy within the metabolism so it can be used if absolutely necessary.

In general, this will allow the control of the visceral organs that exist beneath the diaphragm, which is primarily the digestive tract. It manages the ability to digest food, as well as the freezing that you may see when under stress. When you see a person freeze, there is a good chance that they are using their dorsal vagal complex to respond to the stress in their life at that particular moment.

Ventral Vagal Complex

Over time, however, mammals have had plenty of time to develop this part of the brain. The vagus nerve took time and evolution to grow into the nerve that you know today. This came with further functionality and methods of handling stressors around you, such as being able to actually act when exposed to fear.

In particular, the ventral vagal complex is known as the smart vagus in contrast to the dorsal vagal complex's reputation as the vegetative vagus. This is where you are going to start seeing myelination on the nerves, insulating them and helping them to fire quicker than the other areas. The ventral vagal complex begins to activate sympathetic regulation from this area. It can use the parasympathetic response to take away power from the sympathetic fight or flight response, for example.

The behaviors that will primarily be attributed to this area of the brain include social communication and attempts at self-soothing.

Essentially, this complex is capable of regulating and inhibiting or disinhibiting defensive methods that your body uses. It does more than this as well; however, it controls areas such as controlling the visceral organs above the diaphragm, such as the heart and lungs, as well as impacting the esophagus, bronchi, pharynx, and the larynx. This allows for the vagus nerve to be able to, but is a sort of limiting factor, over the heart's pace at any given point of time. It keeps your heart from beating far quicker than it otherwise would. Your resting heart rate, for example, is the product of your vagus nerve activating and controlling your heart. It slows it down because there is no real reason for the heart to be pumping at full speed when there is no stress around you.

Purpose of the Vagus Nerve

This all happens for very specific reasons; your body has this nerve to regulate many different systems. Let's take a look at some of the primary capabilities of the vagus nerve:

It Grants Sensory Functionality

The vagus nerve specifically allows for certain areas of the body to transmit sensory information. In particular, data about the functionality of your heart, lungs, and digestive tract all go through the vagus nerve. It allows for your body to know how to regulate your breathing, your heart rate, and the digestion of food, allowing it to control when to propel the food from the stomach into the intestines for further digestion.

It Allows For Special Sensory Functions

Special sensory functions are those that are specifically related to your five senses of sight, smell, touch, hearing, and taste. In particular, the vagus nerve innervates an area of the tongue that is responsible for taste at the base of the tongue.

It Allows For Motor Functions to Occur

The vagus nerve also controls your movements in many different areas. Have you ever thought about how much goes into ensuring that you are able to swallow food, for example? Swallowing requires the activation of many different muscles throughout the mouth and neck, and yet we do it effortlessly thanks to the vagus nerve. It regulates these movements that you need to use to eat and speak.

It Regulates Your Parasympathetic Nervous System

Your parasympathetic nervous system is a crucial part of your autonomic functionality. It allows you to cope with the stressors in your environment. In particular, the parasympathetic nervous system is meant to sort of shut off the fight, flight, and freeze response that your body is likely to have when you engage with something that is a cause of concern for you.

What Happens If the Vagus Nerve Is Damaged?

As we have observed, it is possible that the vagus nerve can be damaged. The nerve can be damaged due to excessive pressure on it or due to stress. Continuous stimulation of the nerve can lead to damage if it is not done in the right way. There are also surgical medical procedures that can lead to the nerve being cut or damaged by surgical instruments. In any case, nerve damage can cause serious problems for the patient.

If your nerve is completely damaged, you may experience some of the following problems.

- **Speaking or Voice Problems:** Damaged nerves can affect the voice box, which may lead to a wheezy voice or difficulty in speaking.

- **Trouble Eating and Drinking:** Any damage to the vagus nerve may affect how your throat muscles operate. Given that they are responsible for swallowing food, you will eventually experience problems when taking food or swallowing water. In essence, the vagus nerve damage mainly affects the gag reflex. As we have already observed, the gag reflex is responsible for ensuring that the food pipe is open to allow the swallowing of foods as you eat.

- **Loss of Hearing or Pain in the Ear:** There are high chances that your hearing will be affected in the event of your vagus nerve becoming damaged. Any damage to the vagus nerve may lead to pain in the ear, given that the nerve extends to the outermost part of the ear.

- **Affected Heart Rate and Blood Pressure:** When your vagus nerve is affected, you must expect significant changes in your heart rate and blood pressure. The vagus nerve is the extension of the autonomic nervous system that directly links the heart to the brain.

- **Abdominal Pains and Stomach Pains:** Damage to the vagus nerve often leads to decreased stomach acids. This means that you may experience some problems with food digestion.

Chapter 5: Vagus Nerve and Wellbeing

Vagus Nerve and Fibromyalgia

T here is still not much known about fibromyalgia, as the pain does not come from a specific cause or area in the body. Many researchers believe that with fibromyalgia, painful sensations are amplified due to the way the brain processes pain. A real reason is not fully known regarding this issue.

Sometimes the pain is triggered by a particular event, like an accident or surgery. Other times, there is no single experience, but the pain just seems to accumulate over time. There is no cure for fibromyalgia at this moment. However, there are interventions, both medical and nonmedical, that can help with subsiding the symptoms that come with it. Once again, our friend, the vagus nerve, is at play here.

In a 2011 NIH study, the leading researchers suggested that the vagus nerve stimulation may be a useful adjunct treatment for fibromyalgia patients. Further research was definitely needed, though. Many researchers feel that the vagus nerve stimulation is effective in treating pain because it is able to negate a wide variety of factors that contribute to pain, like inflammation and the pain response. There is still much that is up in the air about fibromyalgia. However, the results of studies continue to suggest that the pain associated with it is significantly reduced with vagus nerve stimulation. Pain is often heightened during times when the body is at stress. Since the vagus nerve can lower a person's stress through the sympathetic response, it is reasonable to believe it can reduce or even eliminate pain associated with fibromyalgia.

Vagus Nerve and Epilepsy

We have been mentioning epilepsy or seizure disorder throughout this portion of the book. Namely, because it was the primary disorder that was targeted by the vagus nerve stimulation for being able to be cured with the proper techniques. Furthermore, many positive benefits of the vagus nerve stimulation were discovered while the researchers were studying the effects of it with epilepsy. Epilepsy is a major central nervous disorder in which brain activity becomes exceedingly abnormal, causing seizures or periods of a very unusual behavior. The nerves and neurons are firing uncontrollably, causing erratic and uncontrollable movements. A person who has epilepsy has their whole world turned upside down due to the severity of the condition and the way it takes over their life. A person will often never know when a seizure will hit, which can prevent them from doing many activities like driving. It will also inhibit their ability to go into certain professions. It is a dangerous and stressful disease to have to deal with.

During an epileptic episode, the sympathetic nervous system is incomplete overdrive, causing excessive and erratic movements within the nervous system. When a person is having a full-blown epileptic attack or seizure, we probably won't be able to attempt the many stimulating practices we went over. Much more extreme measures will need to be taken. However, what can be done is the vagal tone can be strengthened to help avoid or reduce epileptic attacks in the future. The stronger the vagal tone, the better adept the parasympathetic response will be, and the better it will become at inhibiting the sympathetic response. We mentioned before how massaging the carotid sinus has been shown to inhibit seizure activity by stimulating the vagus nerve. If this technique can work, then it is a good indication that the other methods will also.

The overall goal is to continuously improve and strengthen the vagus nerve as much as possible. We will not be able to prevent or cure all illnesses. However, as we maintain our own vagal tone, we can help to improve the functionality of the body and at least prevent or reduce many diseases. The point of the vagus nerve stimulation is to keep it healthy, active, and strong, so that it has the ability to enhance parasympathetic activity as much as possible. When we increase our body's ability to utilize the parasympathetic response, we will be able to reduce seizure activity effectively.

Most of the research behind the vagus nerve stimulation has been to help prevent epilepsy. This suggests that it is still considered a strong therapy in inhibiting seizure activity.

Anxiety and Vagus Nerve

Nervousness can be a genuine doozy; it's outlandishly muddled, profoundly close to home, and ridiculously difficult to foresee. There are times when we think our uneasiness is behind us; that we are at long last one stage ahead, yet then something happens and we are on our heels once more, battling to return to a position of harmony and quiet. We are on the whole understudies of our uneasiness, and that is the reason, seeing precisely, how our sensory system functions, and what we can do to quiet it can be staggeringly enabling.

In any case, what does 'quietening your sensory system' truly mean? Numerous individuals would depict it as easing back the pulse, developing the breath, and loosening up various muscles, however, what really associates these sensations to the mind? You need to know more about the vagus nerve, the piece of the body that appears to clarify how our psyches control our bodies, how our bodies impact our brains, and may give us the instruments we have to quieten them both.

Posttraumatic stress issues (PTSD) are encountered by numerous individuals. Ongoing catastrophic events, mass shootings, psychological oppressor assaults, and urban communities under attack add to the worldwide weight of PTSD which, as indicated by a recent report, influences 4–6% of the worldwide populace, despite the fact that most of injuries are identified with mishaps and sexual or physical savagery. Shockingly, there is no known fix, and flow medicines are not powerful for all patients.

A PTSD psychopharmacology working group as of late, distributed their accord proclamation calling for a quick activity to address the emergency in PTSD treatment, referring to three significant concerns. To start with, just two medications (sertraline and paroxetine) are endorsed by the US FDA for the treatment of PTSD. These meds decrease the side effect's seriousness, however may not create total reduction of the side effects. The subsequent concern is identified with polypharmacy. PTSD patients are recommended prescriptions to address every one of their numerous extraordinary and assorted side effects, including nervousness, trouble dozing, sexual brokenness, wretchedness and interminable torment, with lacking exact examinations of medication communications. The high comorbidity among PTSD and fixation gives further difficulties to pharmacotherapies. The third significant concern is the absence of headways in the treatment of PTSD; no new prescriptions have been endorsed since 2001.

Going past the side effect alleviation, the 'best quality level' injury centered way to deal with treating PTSD pathology is an introduction-based treatment, where patients are presented the tokens of the injury until they figure out how to connect these prompts with wellbeing. In spite of the fact that there is great proof for adequacy with this methodology, not all patients completely react to the treatment. Introduction treatment relies upon stifling the adapted dread memory, which is overwhelmed by another memory that is created through rehashed exposures. The patients with a nervousness issue and PTSD show weaknesses in their capacity to quench adapted feelings of dread, which may meddle with the advancement in treatment. Since the memory of the injury isn't lost at the same time, it rather upgrades through treatments that rely upon new learned affiliations that rival horrible affiliations; the parity of the two recollections can move after some time, prompting backslide. Different difficulties incorporate the trouble in perceiving and smothering apprehension of every single molded boost, and a high dropout rate, which isn't astonishing given that shirking is one of the indications of PTSD.

The Vagus Nerve and Stress

Stress is a natural way of reaction to change that the body has to go through. A person is stressed when they face conflicting thoughts or when they feel threatened. If you are in a situation where you think that your life is in danger, you are likely to experience stress. Stress is accompanied by varied physical, emotional, and mental responses. When you are afraid of something or worried about something, the body will prompt specific actions to take place naturally.

Although stress is a normal part of life, it brings varied ups and downs. It is not possible to take care of your nerves if you are always afraid. As a matter of fact, any time stress kicks in, and you should let the nervous system take full control. You may experience pressure from your thoughts, your body, or the environment. In either case, the vagus nerve will directly be affected.

If you are always stressed, the chances are that you may continuously keep on hurting your vagus nerve. We have seen that chronic inflammation only occurs after a long time of natural rehabilitation. If the body keeps on trying to rehabilitate worn-out tissues due to injuries, it will eventually lead to inflammation. The same case applies to stress. If you continuously experience stress, you are likely to stimulate the vagus nerve to such an extent that it is impossible to recover. But how exactly does body stress relate to the vagus nerve?

Any time you are under stress, you suffer from anxiety or panic attacks. Although the symptoms of either anxiety or panic attacks are not visible, it is clear that people who suffer stress may experience some form of anxiety. The brain is programmed to respond to such stressful situations by producing CRF hormones. Although the brain naturally produces such hormones, stressful situations lead to an increased production of these hormones. The CRFs travel through the hypothalamus to the pituitary glands, where they cause the release of another hormone, known as ACTH. This hormone consequently travels through the bloodstream to the adrenal glands. This leads to the stimulation of cortisol and adrenal reaction, which helps protect the boy from stress. As you can see, this process of stress protection is long and directly affects your vagus nerve. When we are suffering from stress, we are likely to get deep into a state of depression if the vagus nerve and the brain get overwhelmed.

Stress and depression have all been linked with an inflammatory brain response. In other words, the process of responding to stress puts the brain under extreme pressure, leading to injuries and inflammation. In other cases, the same applies to the vagus nerve. As the nerve is exposed to the stress of trying to deal with the anxious situation, it is common for the nerve to experience injuries.

Such injuries attract the natural healing process of the body, which eventually results in inflammation. Even though the body naturally fights injuries, continued stress can lead to the constant production of hormones, which ultimately leads to actions that may cause stress to the vagus nerve.

Chronic stress can also lead to an increase in the production of glutamate in the brain. The output of glutamate may directly affect the brain and, as a result, affect the vagus nerve. For instance, glutamate is a neurotransmitter that causes migraines and depression when produced in excess. When you are under stress, it is common for the brain to initiate the production of this neurotransmitter. To protect yourself from such conditions and to ensure that you preserve your vagus nerve from any damage, ensure that you reduce stressful moments in your life. There are many ways of dealing with stress, including meditation, singing, dancing, among others. Such options will help you deal with stress and reduce the pressure on your brain. By acting to reduce pressure on your head, you respond to protect the brain and the vagus nerve as a whole.

All the factors that affect your brain are also impactful to your vagus nerve. Stress does not only change your mind, but it also affects your nervous system. The vagus nerve may completely fail if you keep on undergoing episodes of stress on a daily basis. The inflammation of the vagus nerve may further lead to other health complications. Swelling means that the nerve is not functioning to the maximum. A simple problem, such as inflammation, may lead to digestive and hearing problems. If the case advances, the entire vagus nerve may be affected and hence affect the autonomic nervous system.

Blood Pressure and Heart Rate

Another factor that may lead to the inflammation of the vagus nerve is blood pressure. The human body is designed to maintain a certain level of blood flow. This means that there must be a signal transmission from the heart to the brain that coordinates the blood flow. The flow of the blood depends on the heart rate and the constriction of blood vessels. If the blood vessels are constricted, the heart will be forced to pump the blood a lot faster so as to achieve equal distribution of blood to all body parts. In the same way, if the blood vessels are lost, the heart rate has to reduce to some extent. The vagus nerve is at the center of all the operations that affect the functioning of the heart.

Vagus nerve stimulation devices have been used for various medical purposes for more than 30 years. These devices are either implanted or used externally. Some of the joint implants are devices that range from 1 to 3.5 mA. These devices are mainly designed to influence the heart rate and blood pressure. Some of the diseases that these devices aim to control include epilepsy and heart diseases. With that said, it is evident that the stimulation of the vagus nerve has a significant effect on the blood pressure and the heart rate.

Research shows that most of the devices used in the vagus nerve stimulation, either use mechanical pressure application, or automated electromagnetic waves. In the early 1800s, the data collected from such devices was vital in evaluating the overall health of the vagus nerve. Data such as the Electrocardiogram (ECG), heart rate (HR), and blood pressure (BP) were all evaluated. However, the focus of the modern-day medical applications tend to be on the performance of the device rather than the wellbeing of the nerve. Over the years, most device manufacturers have opted to design invasive devices that do not give out data as it was initially. This does not mean that the devices used for the vagus nerve stimulation are defective in any way. The main concern would be a case where the device was causing overstimulation, resulting in fatigue and injuries to the nerve.

If you choose to use a device that regulates your blood pressure, you must ensure that it does not go beyond the required. Overstimulation of the vagus nerve will obviously lead to excessive production of some enzymes. The parasympathetic activities of the nerve are awakened during a moment when the body should be acting in the opposite direction. Although the ultimate result of reducing the heart rate may be achieved, it is still expensive and painful to experience some complications associated with the stimulation. If you want to stimulate your vagus nerve for the sake of reducing blood pressure and heart rate, only do it selectively. It should not be something you do daily.

Vagus Nerve Stimulation to Heal from Trauma

The body experiences other distressing signs of post-traumatic stress: a tightness in the abdomen, a sinking sensation in the stomach, a familiar pain in the mouth, or a constant sense of fatigue. We now understand that as a part of the recovery process we have to turn to the body and as a result, we have seen an increase in the use of meditation, mindfulness, tai chi, qigong, Feld ink circle, massage, Craniosacral therapy, dietary therapy, and acupuncture for post-traumatic stress disorder.

Such mind-body treatments are helping us to be less passive, less aggressive, and less impulsive to stress. We're growing our understanding of the options we need to make us stay grounded and relaxed. We felt more in need of this. One way the mental-body treatments operate is by activating the vagus nerve. Awareness of how this nerve works offers a profound understanding of traumatic stress and promotes our healing capacity. The vagus nerve has, therefore, taken center stage in the treatment of trauma.

Moreover, mental-body treatments are successful as they require structural improvements in the autonomic nervous system as determined by the increase in the vagus nerve activity. The vagus nerve reaches through the muscles of the nose, inner ear, chest, back, lungs, stomach, and intestines from the brainstem down. Mind-body treatments make changes in how we relate to our surroundings by encouraging a gentle look, and allowing us to try new breathing or activity patterns that communicate specifically with other parts of the body. Researchers also calculate the changes that exist in the vagus nerve, which is often referred to as the respiratory sinus arrhythmia by heart rate variability (HRV). HRV refers to the rhythmic heart rate oscillations that arise with the breath. It's a function of the intervals between beats in the heart. Higher variability in the heart rate is associated with a better ability to withstand or rebound from stress.

Chronic Fatigue and the Vagus Nerve

At the end of the day, if you find that you are suffering from chronic fatigue, your vagus nerve may be the suspect at hand, and that is good news. You can activate your vagus nerve regularly in hopes of getting out of this sort of negative loop where you are too fatigued to get your vagus nerve functioning properly, which then leads you to struggle to function further. Essentially, you need to figure out how to get yourself back into the proper parasympathetic state, and the fatigue will begin to go away on its own.

However, sometimes, the reason that you feel fatigued in general is that you are either finding yourself in constant sympathetic activation, even if only mildly, or you find that you are teetering on the verge of a parasympathetic shutdown. Either of these situations could directly lead you to feel fatigued and unable to cope with the situation at hand.

It's long been known that chronic fatigue syndrome can be triggered by viral infections, and that a non-stop immune response may result in the devitalizing fatigue associated with it. For many years, experts in the medical field believed that it is a person's individual susceptibility that gives birth to the ecology for a particular disease state to take form. Regardless, there are many who thought that the vagus nerve plays a role in the chronic fatigue syndrome, as well as a number of other common health problems. The scientist Michael B. VanElzakker, in particular, argued that chronic fatigue syndrome is a result of the infection of the vagus nerve.

Every time an immune cell detects an infection, it releases cytokines, which promotes inflammation. These substances are detected by the vagus nerve receptors, which in turn signals the brain to activate fatigue, along with myalgia, fever, cold, flu, bacterial infection, and depression. According to VanElzakker, symptoms of chronic fatigue are the same as those of normal sickness, except they are prolonged and are somewhat triggered whenever a bacterium or virus infects the vagal ganglia. The cells activated by the intrusion can attack the vagus nerve by releasing cytokines and other substances that initiate sickness symptoms. This theory proposes that the primary cause of chronic fatigue syndrome is the infection of the vagus nerve.

Obesity and the Vagus Nerve

The brain may relate how hungry or full you are, but at the end of the day, the vagus nerve is the part of the body that tells the stomach what the brain says. The brain functions as a sort of processor for the body, but if the vagus nerve is sending the wrong signals down to the stomach, you may find that you feel hungrier. You may find that the messages of having enough in your stomach never make it up to the brain, or that they are skewed in some other way.

Because the vagus nerve makes up the gut-brain axis in which the stomach and the brain are able to communicate, it can directly be implicated when something goes wrong. Whether something is failing to activate properly due to something else happening, or it is realizing that your body needs more blood sugar due to some other cause, the vagus nerve may very well be at fault.

When it comes to obesity, often it happens due to some sort of dysfunctional relationship with food. Of course, there are always instances in which a hormone leads to weight gain, but for the vast majority of people, that is not the case. Actually, the fact that there is overeating and not enough exercise occurring, and that can be a problem. As the years go on, more and more of the population becomes obese. In part, this can be due to the fact that we do not have to be as active anymore. We do not have to run around to make sure that we can meet all of your needs because we don't have to hunt. You do not have to make sure that you are able to fight off animals or are capable of defending your family to the same degree that you once did, and because of that you may find that at the end of the day you are actually growing complacent. You are busy with work, so you do not exercise as much. You are too busy, so you grab a pizza on the way home. You drive everywhere because it is easier. Suddenly, your caloric needs are actually much lower than they would be for a human out in the wild, having to hunt, grow food, and defend his or her home from that hungry bear that is desperate to get in.

Some people, after gaining weight, find that they just cannot lose it no matter how hard they try. For these people, they may end up seeking weight loss surgery, which is invasive and entirely irreversible. When it is done, it is done and there is no turning back. However, studies have found that you can actually use the vagus nerve to aid in weight loss. In particular, the vagus nerve can be blocked. In blocking the vagus nerve, the individual is then much more likely to feel full for longer. This means that the individual will not be overeating if the vagus nerve gets the wrong message.

In particular, this was found effective. In a clinical trial involving 233 people with BMIs of 35 or over, those who got the experimental generator activated lost roughly 8.5% more body weight over a year than their peers who did not get the shocks. In particular, roughly half of the patients in this experimental group found that they lost up to 20% of their excess weight while another 38% lost 25% of that excess weight. On the other hand, the patients that did not get the shocks during this time found that only 32.5% lost 20% of their weight, and only 23.4% lost 25%.

This shows that there is some degree of promise by using the vagus nerve to curb appetite in order to alleviate obesity without having to remove a portion of the stomach.

Autoimmune Disorders and the Vagus Nerve

Autoimmune disorders are debilitating for those who have to suffer from them. In particular, when you have an autoimmune disorder, you are more likely to be struggling and suffering from all sorts of long-term disorders that are going to slowly, but surely wear down your body. Some of them can be fatal in some instances, diabetes, for example, can lead to major fluctuations in blood sugar that then leads to death if not regulated properly. Others can cause all sorts of other problems, restricting movement or making life incredibly difficult. Others still may try to attack the nervous system, eating away at the important myelin sheathing that is used to ensure the functionality of the brain and nerves.

No matter what autoimmune disorder you suffer from, there is a good chance that you are struggling with your vagus nerve. In particular, you may find that your immune system is too active, leading to a problem with the body attacking itself. That is a problem; when your vagus nerve is not active enough, the body's immune system is free to send out as many cytokines as it wants. In sending out all of these cytokines, you'll find that your body is not going to function properly. Your body will be suppressing your appetite. You will be tired. You will ache.

Beyond that, however, your body will be able to attack whatever it decides it needs to attack. Some autoimmune disorders attack joints, such as rheumatoid arthritis. Others attack other areas of the body. In type 1 diabetes, the cells in the body that create insulin are damaged and destroyed, leading to someone being unable to regulate blood sugar without insulin from elsewhere.

These sorts of autoimmune diseases can lead to all sorts of problems for anyone suffering from them. Thankfully, through the stimulation of the vagus nerve, inflammation, and therefore, autoimmune responses are impeded. When you use your vagus nerve, the body will destroy the proteins that are being used to facilitate all of that communication to create all of the autoimmune problems within it. Essentially, you will find that you are more capable of managing your immune system, or at least, your body will be more capable of managing and regulating your immune system if you ensure that it is managed well through the use of toning your vagus nerve.

Gastroparesis and the Vagus Nerve

In particular, gastroparesis is the result of your body not being able to process food. You will try to push food through your stomach, only to find that you cannot. This is because the vagus nerve, the nerve that is responsible for ensuring that your stomach contracts to allow for the passage of food in the first place, becomes inactive for some reason or another. When that happens, you run into all sorts of problems. You may, for example, find that you struggle to pass food, which leads to all sorts of other problems along the way.

When you cannot pass food, it can do one of the three things: you can vomit it up to get it out of your stomach; it can be left in the stomach to ferment and make you sick; or it can harden in your stomach and further block the passage of food. Obviously, none of these are very good choices. You would not want to suffer from any of these effects.

When the vagus nerve has been disrupted or otherwise, it is just not working properly, the end result can be that your stomach never does pass the food, or it may do so sporadically. This means that the body will not be able to regulate out its own ability to process food and blood sugar; you may find that your blood-sugar tanks because you cannot take in any of the carbohydrates that you would use to turn into glucose. You may find that your blood sugar suddenly spikes when food is allowed to pass through the body, completely unregulated. The body will simply struggle to really process its food, and that can be a major problem for you. You need to eat, and you need nourishment.

If the gastroparesis is due to an injury that has severed the vagus nerve, there is not really any fix for you at this point in time. However, if it is because your vagus nerve is acting up and you know you have not had surgery or injuries that could potentially harm your vagus nerve, you may find that you are best served by getting it tested. How much can you stimulate it? Can you activate it more to tone it? When you tone it, you may find that it gets better at regulating your digestive system, so you know that you can actually process the food that you have to take in.

Vagus Nerve and Inflammation

Inflammation is significant for making sure you respond to different stimuli within the body correctly. With inflammation, you have either an injury, or a pain, or even an infection, and from this, you get more white blood cells, immune cells, and cytokines that are used for curing the disease.

Inflammation is something that should be short-term, with redness, heat, swelling, and pain. But, in some cases, you might have inflammation happening within the body; without symptoms, you usually don't notice.

When there is something in the body that the brain recognizes as an invader, it starts the inflammation in the body. However, when not properly turned off, it can cause a lot of problems.

Well, anything that yields an inflammatory response is a culprit here. For example, diabetes, heart disease, cancer, fatty liver disease, asthma, Chron's disease, IBS, and pretty much anything with inflammation, as the cause is a part of this.

Food allergies and sensitivities are also seen here. Insulin resistance is another symptom of inflammation, hence this is why type 1 diabetes is often a result of inflammation in the body.

While some of the inflammation can be turned off quite quickly, you'll realize that, with every single stimulus, it can actually make a lot of issues for people, and it can have a lot of problems that are very hard to fix if you're not careful.

People who are obese, or under a lot of stress, usually there is chronic inflammation there.

While you might notice it most of the time, you have to see a doctor and get some blood tests done, including the C-reactive protein test, TMF alpha, and the IL-6, all of which are different chemicals that are within the body whenever you have an inflammatory response.

Well, there are many different causes here, and the vagus nerve is actually a part of this. When the vagus nerve is stimulated correctly, it sends out the neurotransmitters to tell the inflammatory response that it's over, the invader is gone, and you don't need to activate, which causes a reduced reaction.

But, with a vagus nerve that's improperly stimulated, it can cause you to have an overstimulation of the inflammatory response within the body, resulting in insulin resistance, heart disease, obesity, and also other conditions.

This is partially caused by your diet, of course. Eating high amounts of sugars, carbs, high fructose corn syrup, and consuming a diet that's riddled with junk food is a part of the reason why you might have inflammatory responses, and the solution, in that case, is, of course, a diet change.

If you're stressed, and continuously activating the parasympathetic nervous system, your vagus nerve will be affected too. This, in turn, causes an inflammatory response in the body also, and hence, diseases will come forth too.

But, it's more than just the sugars. It's also how your vagus nerve is stimulated. When your vagus nerve isn't working, it won't control the inflammatory response, and oftentimes won't control the signals to the brain. This will, in turn, lead to debilitating conditions in the boy as we've tackled before.

In many instances, when we're continually reducing our 'flight or fight' responses, the biological markers will help with reducing inflammation.

When you see a doctor for inflammation, chances are that they won't prescribe medications for that. That's because the way to combat inflammation can't always be handled with medication, and oftentimes, drugs cause more side effects than help to the body.

The vagus nerve affects your heart rate, and also acetylcholine, which is a tranquilizer that you can administer to yourself through merely inhaling and exhaling, and from there, your parasympathetic nervous system will be activated.

When you activate this, you're essentially encouraging the 'rest and digest' or the 'tend and befriend' actions in the body. The 'tend and befriend' actions within your organization, of course, are those neurotransmitters that are activated.

When you activate your vagus nerve, you're basically turning off all of those responses you don't need in the body, and it'll help with inflammation.

The Vagus Nerve and the Phobias

People often hear about or experience others being afraid of certain things, and that's not necessarily worrisome but when it grows fiercer and intense, it's definitely something to be worried about. The fear from a certain thing, situation or an entity when it grows stronger, is deemed as a phobia. There are many types of phobias and they are all intense no matter which kind. Also, they're impossible to escape because it's an unavoidable facet of human life. But hey! Don't bite your nails out of fear now! The vagus nerve has the solution to your problem, but prior to jumping in, let's find out the biological presence of phobia in a human brain and its types (of course, not all of them!).

Phobia unlike fear is not a rush of terror that just passes away when the horror movie ends. These are mental disorders that even doctors diagnose in patients. The patients when they come in contact with what triggers their phobia either freeze, get a panic attack, forget to breath and face intense distress, or in some cases they die from a heart attack. Yes, it's that serious! Now, what causes phobia?

It often starts in childhood; it could be acquired from a parent or a family member. Also, some events can cause this, such as a near death experience involving an object or an entity, which then begins to haunt them for a lifetime. It could be a drowning experience where they got lucky and were saved in time, or it could be a terrifying or traumatic event involving darkness. It could be anything, and there are no specific causes. Now, when the brain witnesses all of that, it stores it somewhere and then replays it in the mind after being triggered to do so; that is when the object, situation or an entity they are afraid of appears in front of them. These chemical reactions take place in the amygdala which causes the stress to overpower the patient, and they then feel intense fear surfacing, namely their phobia. Now, let's discuss its symptoms.

Our vagus nerve is joined to our brain from one end to the other, and to all the organs of the body. Basically, it is the one that commands the brain to execute orders. Therefore, when the panic rises and the phobia is triggered, the vagus nerve is stimulated and causes the fight or flight response to emerge. This helps the person get out of the situation quicker by fighting it or flying from it. Therapists make use of certain techniques to stimulate the vagus nerve in these people. They deliberately let the patients face what they fear and have a phobia of. With this exposure, they instruct the patient to take deep breaths which stimulates the vagus nerve. The therapists also ask the patient to sit back and relax, which is also a vagus nerve stimulator.

The Vagus Nerve and Irritable Bowel Syndrome

Irritable bowel syndrome or IBS is a very troublesome disease. It involves altered bowel habits such as:

- Bloating

- Gas

- Diarrhea

- Chronic constipation

- Severe pain and discomfort in the abdomen

This disease is not necessarily a serious one or known to be 'life threatening,' but the symptoms keep the person troubled and causes unrest to develop in their mind. The bi-directional interaction between the gut and the brain creates a brain-gut axis which keeps the balance maintained in the gastrointestinal tract. The main cause of this disease is still not discovered, but a few sources say that Irritable Bowel Syndrome is usually caused by certain allergies, stress (either physical or mental) and at times, it has been reported to be transferred from a parent. The changes in one's lifestyle, environment and other areas are responsible in contributing in the occurrence of IBS. But there is a cure to IBS that would help you get rid of it with little effort. Want to know what? What are you waiting for then? Let's dive in!

Get your vagus nerve examined for damage and see if its dysfunction is causing IBS to occur, since it is the pathway between the gut and the brain that deals with all the aspects of the gastrointestinal tract. If they fail to find any damage, seek to activate the vagus nerve to maintain the vagal tone index as that does all the work. The vagus nerve communicates with the brain about the problems occurring and the brain jumps into action to solve all the issues including bloating, gas, abdominal pain and other symptoms IBS brings. The stomach acid runs low during IBS and the vagus nerve makes sure that this doesn't happen by causing the cells to release histamines which creates the stomach acid that the body needs to break the food down. Now, when the vagus nerve is activated through various ways, where the non-invasive transcutaneous vagus nerve stimulation and deep belly breathing along with some exercise is mostly preferred, it provides various other benefits such as:

- Promotes relaxation

- Balances heart rate

- Eradicates anxiety

- Alleviates depression

- Controls blood pressure

Plus, many other countless benefits occur when one keeps the health of their vagus nerve in check and makes sure that it is stimulating normally, and effectively eradicating all the troubles that come their way. Well, it doesn't end here, there is more to the vagus nerve that you need to unveil!

Vagus Nerve and Depression

When people think of mental health issues, the two that come to mind are typically anxiety and depression. Depression is the other most common mental health issue around the world, and many people suffer from it. It is estimated that somewhere around 15% of the people will experience depression, either acute or chronic, at some point in their lives.

This disorder can be debilitating. It can be exhausting. It can be draining, and it can be destructive. It can lead to so many different problems, and that can be a primary reason you would benefit from trying to solve the problem altogether. Instead of continuing to stress about the issue, you can defeat the problem.

Depression itself is the feeling of negativity and hopelessness that people sometimes feel. It is a period in which there is a lack of interest in the world around you. You can feel like you do not want to engage with other people. You find that anything you used to be interested in is no longer compelling. You do not want to do anything at all oftentimes, and that can sometimes really just make the problem worse.

Depression can be debilitating for these people. Especially when severe, people who suffer from depression can find they do not have the energy for anything at all. They feel slow, sleepy, even if they cannot sleep, they feel stuck and unhappy. Even the activities that once brought them joy in life are no longer enjoyable, and they find that they cannot do anything about it. This is a significant problem for people; it can really hold them back.

Remember, when the body feels that something is entirely futile, it shuts itself off; it stops trying to continue moving forward. It finds there is no reason to stay, so it begins to shut down and slow down. When you go into a frozen state, this is what happens. Your body dulls your mind, and you struggle to concentrate. You lose interest and responsiveness. You feel like you cannot move at all, or like moving or doing anything at all would take far too much effort out of your life.

The vagus nerve, when it is overactive, can trigger what is known as a parasympathetic shutdown. This is the freeze response. It is a primitive response to fear, developed long before mammals developed their more modern, nuanced fight or flight system. It is believed that depression, at or at least, certain kinds of depression, may be linked to this.

There are many types of depression that can be found to be resistant to just about all treatment options; these people are known to have treatment-resistant depression, and yet, stimulating the vagus nerve has been shown to help these people begin to get back to their old routine.

It may also be the case that depression is related to inflammation, especially if the swelling is treated when you stimulate the vagus nerve. Nevertheless, regardless of whether depression is caused in the same way that anxiety is, one thing is known for sure; depression can be managed with the stimulation of the vagus nerve.

We are going to consider three methods that you can use to begin fighting off depression. We are going to look at probiotics; these are relevant to the vagus nerve thanks to the prominent role that the vagus nerve plays in the digestive system and the digestive system's leading role in the production of serotonin, which happens to be one of the ways that we can treat depression. We will take a look at socialization to help bring the vagus nerve back to a sense of normalcy, and finally, we will take a look at meditation.

Vagus Nerve and PTSD

Post-Traumatic Stress Disorder, or PTSD, is a mental condition caused by a traumatic event that had a severe impact on someone. The people who are most commonly affected are in the military, the law enforcement, or are the first responders, or anyone in a field where tragedy is a common occurrence. However, PTSD may also strike just about anybody and everybody who has been through a traumatic event. A serious accident, death of a loved one, getting assaulted, or any number of tragic events may cause a person to have PTSD. It may take years to overcome PTSD, and some never overcome it at all. PTSD can manifest itself in multiple ways, including anxiety, anger, nervousness, negative thoughts, flashbacks, and chronic pain. They will often re-experience the trauma various times in their heads. There is a significant split, even within the military community, whether or not PTSD is legitimate.

For this reason, just like with depression, people will dismiss it as a non-issue. They believe that someone can just get over it. A person cannot only get over it, though.

PTSD is genuine and is a severe mental disorder that needs to be treated as such. Unfortunately, PTSD continues to carry a negative stigma to it that can hopefully be a thing of the past once people start realizing some of the physical elements to it as well.

While there is no known cure for PTSD, there are therapies that may be used to help subside some of the signs and symptoms. Currently, some of the treatments include talk therapy and exposure therapy. Several studies suggest that the vagus nerve stimulation may be a productive adjunct therapy for helping with PTSD, especially with its associated pain. A University of Texas, Dallas, researched the effects of the vagus nerve stimulation on rats. The rats in this particular study were shown to display some signs that come with PTSD, like fear, aggression, and anxiety. A session of vagus nerve stimulation showed a significant reduction in these negative signs. Not only that, but the symptoms also did not return in many cases after another episode of trauma, suggesting that the stimulation may have more long-term effects than the other therapies. Researchers feel that if the stimulus can work in the same manner in humans, it may significantly reduce the pain associated with PTSD.

If the effects are more long term as well, it is undoubtedly an adjunct therapy worth looking into.

If you have a friend or loved one who experiences PTSD, perhaps it is time to work on them. Help them by using the techniques that will stimulate their vagus nerve. That old cliché of *laughter is the best medicine* may be the ultimate tool. Help your loved one get regular exercise. Remember, this does not just mean going to the gym. Most people are more likely to do something if they enjoy it. Find something they want to do physically and help them do it. If they love playing basketball, play a quick pickup game. If they love going for walks, find a beautiful trail, and enjoy the sites. Whatever you can do to get them moving, do it. Finally, how about a nice round of karaoke? Singing and dancing are a great way to stimulate the vagus nerve and get your friends out of the poor mental state. If we can continue to correlate the vagus nerve stimulation with helping to subside the signs of PTSD, we can hopefully remove the stigma associated with it. Just like with depression, we may never be able to cure PTSD, but we can certainly manage it with the appropriate practices.

We want to talk about how PTSD can manifest itself into physical symptoms like muscle tightness, chest pain, fatigue, and digestive issues. Many of these physical responses to a traumatic event indicate a sympathetic nervous system activity. Things like muscle tightness and chest pain that is not heart-related, often come from stress and being worked up for so long. They do not come from being in a relaxed state. Furthermore, fatigue develops when the body is overly stressed for long periods. This is why excessive sympathetic responses are not healthy for the organization. If your body is in a constant state of pain and tiredness due to a traumatic event, then perhaps it is time to stimulate your vagus nerve to inactivate your parasympathetic response. The parasympathetic response inhibition will put your body in a state of relaxation, releasing the built-up tension and helping reduce the pain associated with PTSD. Do this regularly, and it can help to manage the negative signs and symptoms of the post-traumatic stress disorder.

The Vagus Nerve and Chronic Pancreatitis

Chronic pancreatitis is a part of the inflammation diseases, and it is also connected with the gut. The pancreas is situated right behind the stomach and is responsible for producing special protein enzymes that help the food to be digested. Moreover, the pancreas also controls the level of sugar in the blood by secreting certain hormones.

Now, chronic pancreatitis occurs when inflammation occurs in the pancreas. There are two types of pancreatitis: acute, lasting for a few days, usually does not come back, and chronic pancreatitis, which occurs when the inflammation fails to be eliminated and keeps returning. Also, atop that, it lasts for months and years and keeps growing severe. Chronic pancreatitis causes permanent damage to the pancreas.

The stones of calcium and also the cysts might occur in it too. This would cause blockage to appear in the pancreas, which would prevent the digestive enzymes and fluid from being transferred to the stomach. The stomach would then have trouble digesting the food and regulating the level of sugar in the blood, and keeping diabetes at bay. Also, it usually occurs in people aging from 30 to 40.

The vagus nerve carries the sensory information to the CNS (Central Nervous System). The vagus nerve is a pathway basically where the bi-directional flow of information occurs from the gut to the brain, and then from the brain to the gut. Hence, when chronic pancreatitis occurs, it ultimately knows that it has to send signals to the brain regarding the occurrence of chronic pancreatitis. The pain during this condition is unbearable, and the patient has to take a painkiller.

Vagus Nerve and Migraines

The vagus nerve can be used to help eliminate or reduce migraines significantly. The best part is, we all have a vagus nerve and can use it. It is not certainly known whether the vagus nerve stimulation can definitely help with migraines because that field is not entirely explored. However, several research studies show that people who received the vagus nerve stimulation over multiple years reported a significant improvement in their migraines. This also happened in the frequency and pain level.

A survey conducted by Southern Illinois University for individuals who received the vagus nerve stimulation for epilepsy showed that multiple people who had migraines before the therapy reported vast improvements in the frequency and pain levels. All of the people who did have migraines before the treatments report vast improvements afterwards. This is a strong indication that the vagus nerve stimulation significantly, positively impacts migraines. Of course, these simulations were done medically using implanted devices. However, many of the techniques we discussed can still have minor, indirect effects.

Many other prominent studies have shown that the stimulation of the vagus nerve, including the noninvasive approach, significantly reduces migraines for many individuals. This further cements that a direct nerve stimulation is not necessary to help relieve migraines. The reporting in the reduction of pain is done by the patients themselves, which is the strongest indication. If a person states they are not in pain, then they are not in pain. Many of these individuals also reported a higher quality of life due to the lack of pain. When a person has less pain, they are more likely to continue healthy practices as well.

A study done by a prominent neurologist in the early 2000s discusses a patient he had with chronic epileptic seizures. Unfortunately, for whatever reason, the Vagus nerve stimulation did not improve epilepsy. Not every therapy will work for every individual as each human organism is unique in its own way. This was an unfortunate circumstance for this patient.

However, they were surprised to learn that the patient had a significant reduction in his chronic migraines. The patient went under treatment for something else and cured something that he never planned to fix. That is amazing not only for the patient, but also for all the people that seek relief for migraines. This was not the intended result but since it worked, the treatment was partially successful. Researchers are continuing to do further studies on this phenomenon between the vagus nerve and the migraines. It was found by accident as multiple people who were getting treated for seizures using stimulation, surprisingly had an improvement in their migraines and headaches.

The parasympathetic response of the vagus nerve seems to reduce and even eliminate the causes of severe migraines significantly. The parasympathetic response likely inhibits the sympathetic nervous system's overstimulation in these cases, effectively altering the pain response. Vagus nerve stimulation also reduces stress, which can be a trigger for migraines. When the sympathetic nervous system is elevated, stress is increased. When the parasympathetic inhibitory response kicks in, stress, and in turn, pain, is significantly decreased. The next time the migraine hits, try some of the techniques we discussed earlier. Go for a long walk or hit the gym. This may be difficult as exercise will be the last thing on your mind. You can also sit and take some deep breaths, hum, or take a cold shower. Whatever looks right for you at that particular, and at the same time, a complicated moment, try it out! Stimulating and utilizing the full potential of the vagus nerve can vastly improve migraines and improve your quality of life.

Chapter 6: Vagus Nerve Hacking

Exposure to Cold Temperature

A study done on ten healthy people suggested that when the body begins to adjust to very low temperatures, the sympathetic system (fight-or-flight) declines and the parasympathetic system (rest-and-relax) is activated, an event mediated by the vagus nerve. In the study, the subjects were exposed to temperatures of 50°F or 10°C. It's also been found that sudden cold exposure to a temperature of 39°F/4°C can increase the vagus nerve activation in rodents. But while the effects of getting a cold shower on the vagus nerve response have not been investigated that much, a lot of people promote this cooling method.

Singing and Chanting

There is something about singing or chanting that is so calming and relaxing that makes one feel joy. Indeed, one study done on healthy 18-year old teenagers found that singing helps to increase the HRV, or the Heart Rate Variability. HRV has been associated with a higher parasympathetic activity (rest-and-digest), as well as with relaxation and better resilience and adaptability to stress.

The researchers who did the study found that chanting, singing a hymn, singing in an energetic and upbeat manner, and even simply humming increases the Heart Rate Variability, albeit in slightly differing ways. They theorized that singing causes the vagus nerve to send relaxing waves to the rest of the body, promoting wellbeing. One reason, the study says, is that singing requires slower respiration, which affects the heart activity.

Meditation

Meditation has a similar effect on the vagus nerve tone as that of singing and chanting. According to studies, there are three types of meditation that have the potential to stimulate the vagus nerve, albeit indirectly: Om chanting, mindfulness meditation, and loving-kindness meditation. Studies done on the effects of these three types of meditation on vagal function found that they increased the heart rate variability. Some experts suggest that the conscious, deep breathing that comes with meditation and other similar practices is responsible for such effects. Attentive breathing, for instance, is found to have a direct effect on the vagus nerve, as well as the rest-and-digest nervous activity.

Prayer

The habit of praying regularly is just as beneficial to the vagus nerve as meditation. It's not a surprise, too, considering that prayer can be a form of meditation in itself. A study done to test the effects of reciting the rosary prayer has been found to increase the activation of the vagus nerve. It has specifically been observed to improve the cardiovascular rhythms, with the ability to reduce the diastolic blood pressure, as well as enhancing the HRV.

The study says that the reading of one rosary cycle takes about 10 seconds. This causes the reader to breathe at 10-second intervals, and this increases the heart rate variability, and consequently, the vagus nerve function.

Optimism and Social Connection

Most people may take the idea of optimism for granted, but science shows evidence that thinking positive thoughts has a significant effect on wellbeing. It particularly has benefits for the vagus nerve functioning. In a study done on 65 participants, for instance, it was discovered that those who thought positive thoughts towards other people showed an increase in positive emotions, such as serenity, joy, amusement, interest, and most importantly, hope. The psychological and emotional changes were associated with a greater sense of connectedness and to an improvement in the function of the vagus nerve as evidenced by an improved HRV.

Reduced Social Media Use

This one is closely connected with the previous point. In the previous section, it was mentioned that social connection had a strong link to a healthier vagal tone. This is interesting, because increased social connection means reduced screen time, which we know is key to better health. As most studies have proven, if there's one factor to blame in the rise of depression and other mental health problems in this age, it's social media. And perhaps one of the reasons that people were healthier in the past is that they relied on the sympathetic nervous system to initiate cortisol production, as well as other neurobiological responses necessary for hunting, gathering, and defending themselves from enemies. On the other hand, the parasympathetic nervous system may have depended on oxytocin to strengthen the innate drive of early humans to nurture relationships, procreate, and build communities.

Regulated Breathing

We've all been taught the importance of breathing exercises to our health, and yet, most people around the world do not practice deep breathing at all. What's even more ironic is that while breathing is an automatic and rhythmic act of the body, a lot of us have been breathing the wrong way the whole time. Regardless, it's been hypothesized that taking deep and slow breaths can stimulate the vagus nerve and is therefore a crucial prerequisite to better health.

Laughter

A lot of studies have been done to prove that laughter is indeed the best medicine. And indeed, laughter has been found to have a positive impact on the vagal tone. One study, in particular, suggests that laughter is capable of stimulating the vagus nerve, concluding that using laughter as a therapy may be beneficial for health. Yoga laughter, as the study suggested, increased the heart rate variability. However, it also cannot be denied that laughter can result in fainting. Doctors point out that the reason may be that too much laughter can overstimulate the vagus nerve.

Probiotics

The connection between the gut and the brain has been mentioned in this work more than a couple times already, so it wouldn't be a surprise to learn that probiotics can enhance the vagus nerve function. The emerging evidence particularly points to the effect of the gut microbiota on brain health and functioning. While there are not enough clinical trials yet, some animal studies have already explored the potential effects of probiotics on the vagus nerve.

Whole Body Vibration Therapy

Vibration is just another way to massage your body and this has resulted in a number of vibration related therapies that can be of benefit to you. Whole body vibration is one of them.

Vibrational therapy has long been used as a complementary approach to a lot of other treatment methods and there is a lot of anecdotal evidence that suggests that this approach improves the overall mood and feelings of well-being.

Red Light Therapy

Red light therapy is a treatment option that has gained a lot of traction over the past decade. The reason for this has a lot to do with social media. Having said that, the benefits of red light therapy are much the same as vibrational therapy in that that it can produce a feeling of wellness in a person's mind and improve their quality of life.

Massage

Massage has long been known to be an excellent way of improving blood circulation. Based on studies, it's one of the simplest and most sensory ways to improve the vagal tone. Massaging certain areas of the body, such as the carotid sinus located on the neck, in particular, stimulates the vagus nerve. According to one study, this practice may be able to help reduce seizures. Carotid sinus massage, a technique that involves digital pressure on the innervated carotid sinus, is said to be a great method for the termination of supraventricular tachycardia (SVT) as a result of the paroxysmal atrial tachycardia. Recently, vagal nerve stimulation has been found to be a better technique. This technique employs a pacemaker stimulation of the vagus nerve as a treatment for refractory epilepsy. This method can be used to suppress seizures and can result in a therapeutic neurological outcome. This technique shouldn't be done at home, however, as it can result in fainting if not performed correctly.

Not only that, but pressured massage has also been found to activate the vagus nerve and help underweight infants gain weight. Reflexology foot massage, too, is said to be an effective way to increase vagal activity and improve HRV, resulting in a lower heart rate and blood pressure.

Fasting

Intermittent fasting is no new practice, but it wasn't only until Martin Berkhan of **Lean Gains** popularized the term that more people became interested in it. There are different ways to do it, but regardless of how it's done, there are many who say that it can increase heart rate variability just as well as it can reduce calories. Again, HRV is considered a marker of vagal tone, so the higher the HRV level, the healthier the vagus nerve is said to be. No clinical trait can attest to this claim, although some tests have already been done on animals with favorable results.

Enough Sleep

There is no question to the importance of sleep to a person's wellbeing. Science has long been telling us that human beings should be able to get at least eight hours of sleep to remain healthy.

Increased Salivation

The calmer the brain and also the deeper the comfort, the simpler the stimulation of salivation is. The mouth can create copious amounts of spit while you are aware that the vagus nerve was aroused, and the body is in concentric mode. To stimulate salivation, attempt relaxing and relax in a chair and envision a hot lemon.

Since your mouth is filled with saliva, simply put your tongue within this tub (if this does not occur, simply fill your mouth with a small amount of warm water and then put your tongue out within the bathroom. Only the custom of relaxing will trigger the secretion of saliva).

Expressive Journaling

Recent research from the University of Arizona found that 20 minutes of narrative expressive writing on a regular basis can initiate a physiological chain reaction that is linked to improved heart rate variability. This particular study doesn't directly look at the vagus nerve stimulation, but previous studies have shown that an improved HRV is one of the keys to a strong parasympathetic nervous response and a more robust vagal tone, and this keeps the balance between the responses of the parasympathetic and sympathetic nervous systems.

Third-Person Self-Talk

Self-talk is the internal chatter that all people experience. It can either be negative or positive, supportive or self-defeating, and is the brain's way of interpreting and processing experiences that one goes through on a daily basis. In more recent years, a number of studies have come out proving the benefits of positive self-talk. One study, in particular, found that a regular third-person self-talk, whether inside one's head or in a hushed tone, can help optimize the vagus nerve response. Again, heart rate variability is a marker for a healthy vagal tone, and it's been discovered that self-distancing done through a third-person self-talk can have a profound effect on the HRV.

Gargling

Another fun way to stimulate the vagus nerve at home is to gargle with water. This action stimulates the muscles in the soft palate within your mouth which are directly being controlled by the vagus nerve.

You can even spice things up and hum while you are gargling to add to the effect that you will have on your vagus nerve to wake it up. Kids also find this particular kind of exercise most amusing, and they can equally benefit from it being turned into a family game of sorts to see who can gargle the longest or loudest (letting them win will have an equally amusing effect).

Coffee Enemas

Here is one for the not-so faint of heart. Did you know that by having an enema done, you are giving your vagus nerve the workout of a lifetime?

It doesn't sound like fun, but your vagus nerve will love you for it! Enemas are somewhat like a marathon or a 100-meter dash for your vagus nerve. By expanding your bowel with a coffee enema, you are increasing your vagus nerves activation levels.

This deep (please excuse the pun) cleansing of your insides is accomplished by an overall increase in the liver's ability as well as capacity to filter out the toxins in the blood. In the meantime, the liver is also able to cleanse itself of these toxins by releasing bile into the small and large intestines where it is well on its way towards evacuation through your bowels. The total amount of blood in your body is constantly circulating through your liver at a rapid rate of a full cleanse every three minutes.

If you are retaining your coffee enema for up to 15 minutes or longer, the blood in the system is able to circulate through the liver a few times for cleansing, and works much like a dialysis treatment would. The water content of the coffee enema will stimulate the gut into a form of intestinal peristalsis in order to help cleanse and empty the large intestine of any accumulated toxins and bile that have been removed from the system.

Experiencing Awe

It may seem surprising that immersing one in something 'awesome' can benefit the health, but that's just what *awe* can actually do. When we talk about awe, we simply mean the feeling you get when you are in the presence of something that's vast and beyond understanding. There are many factors that can inspire awe. In fact, the spectrum of stimuli is very broad. It can include looking up at the stars at night, being amazed with the brilliant colors of sunset, being immersed in the beauty of the nature, hearing some breathtaking music or laying eyes on some spectacular piece of art.

Kindness

Kindness, whether shown to others or to oneself has been found to tone the vagus nerve. In 2013, research was done to study how loving-kindness meditation or LKM, affected the vagal tone, and how it promoted positive emotions and improved the physical health. The study found that sending loving-kindness towards oneself and towards others, whether a loved one, friend, or enemy, is the key to an improved vagal tone.

Socialization to Stimulate the Vagus Nerve

Once again, we come right back to the social nervous system, the proposed method through which the vagus nerve regulates the way in which we socialize. It has been found that socialization is one of the most significant ways to reduce stress, and this makes sense. Think about it; we are social creatures. If you want to alleviate stress, you need to be around people you love and care about. This socialization can leave you feeling fulfilled and better than ever.

Chapter 7: Vagus Nerve Exercises

E xercise and physical movement challenges you and gives you a sense of accomplishment which directly opposes the miserable feeling that depression causes. In case anxiety is your issue, exercise gives you an opportunity to vent your frustration at something.

Exercise also releases endorphins in your system and helps you feel better. All in all there is no downside to exercise and you should aim to make it a part of your daily routine.

Diaphragmatic Breathing

Most people will inhale up to 14 times per minute and in doing so, have superficial breathing. When you become more self-aware of your breathing rate, you are able to lower the amount to a more ideal breathing rate of 6 inhales per minute.

This forces your body to practice deeper breathing techniques and fill your lungs to capacity with each breath. It's incredibly easy to practice this routine wherever you may be. I'm practicing it right now as I type! This type of breathing exercise, especially helps to trigger the vagus nerve and turns on the full activation as it is telling the brain that it is now necessary to calm down, even though the nerve itself has not been given that particular instruction directly. In this way, the mechanism is the same as when you close your eyes and tap against your eyelids gently. Your brain will perceive each tap as a spark of light shining through.

When we breathe in deeper breaths, we are making use of the lower part of our chests and moving the diaphragm in such a way that it will promote relaxation.

The Power of Stretching

Stretching is used to help naturally stimulate the body and make movement simple. There is a lot you can get from this, and you can get out of this. Most people don't realize that they're not only releasing tension within the muscles when they stretch, but they're also focusing their breathing, so it's simple and yet very useful.

A lot of people don't stretch enough, so that tension sits there. But, a way to naturally start up the parasympathetic nervous system and activate the vagus nerve is to do just this. Sitting down, stretching out your body, and working on this helps promote relaxation and wellness, and from there it will stimulate your entire body in its way.

Try touching your toes, stretching your arms behind your head, pushing them up, and holding your arms in the air, or even just moving towards your foot will help with this. There is a lot of benefits to be had with stretching and a lot of beautiful things to do with this. You'll be shocked, you'll be amazed, and most of all, you'll be quite happy with the power of this small exercise. You'll feel invigorated for whatever is to come for you in the future.

Consider stretching right before you begin your day, or at the end of the night, and see how it helps you feel during the day. You'll feel your vagus nerve stimulated almost immediately.

Weight Training

Weight training might seem weird to do to stimulate the vagus nerve, but it does work. That's because, when you lift weights, it is changing the speed of the body. Plus, through the power of repetition, you get your body to relax. A lot of people think lifting weights is only for big, burly people, but that isn't the case.

Ever just doing a few sets of curls will change the way your body feels, and your vagus nerve. Many people also think they need to start with a heavyweight right away, but that isn't the case.

HIIT Workouts

HIIT, or 'High-Intensity Interval Training' is a form of workouts that require you to do a lot in a minimal period. Sometimes, this involves sprinting; other times, this can be push-ups, sit-ups, or other exercises. The main goal behind this is to do a lot in a bit of time, and through spurts.

These spurts are what cause the vagus nerve stimulation. The vagus nerve is usually not stimulated if you're always stressed out. Still, the periods of stress, and then relaxation, kick the vagus nerve into gear, helping it activate whenever needed.

HIIT workouts are also great because they are often straightforward to do. No matter what it is that you do, you'll feel the difference in these immediately.

Walking

Walking is an excellent option if you're not going to the gym to lift or don't want to spend time doing HIIT or yoga.

Walking is an excellent habit to get into because it stimulates your body and helps with physical fitness and wellness. Your vagus nerve will get stimulated with walking, especially if you live a sedentary lifestyle.

I think walking for 30 minutes a day is ideal, especially if you're unable to do this otherwise. Sometimes, pacing while on your breaks is a great way to do this, and walking also lets you improve on your health and wellness.

You will want to do this to help with your physical fitness, and walking is a good start, especially if you're not active otherwise.

Jogging is also another good one because this can help with deep breathing. A lot of people, when they start, will get into the habit of breathing with short breaths, but that won't work here. This can make it hard to run, and you might pass out. With jogging, you want to make sure that you're breathing in a slow, deep, and even manner, and focus on this. This will help with your vagus nerve and help you get into the habit of breathing deeply. You can also do running with this, but it's more high-intensity and it might be harder to engage in deep breathing otherwise.

Jumping

Again, another form of cardio that's great, but your vagus nerve will love it. Jumping jacks, burpees, and other jumping exercises are useful because they help improve circulation, which can help with blood pressure and your vagal tone.

When you jump too, be mindful of your breathing. Try to do it with a deep breath, and you'll notice it's a much harder workout, but you'll feel the difference. It increases blood flow, blood pressure, and heart rate as well.

Your vagus nerve will thank you for this, and you'll be able to, with jumping too, improve your health and wellness.

Yoga

There's still not a lot of studies done on the effects of yoga on the vagus nerve, but the ones that have been conducted suggest that yoga does increase the vagus nerve activity. For instance, a 12-week yoga intervention was found to be more beneficial in terms of mood improvement than walking exercises. A study conducted on the effects of yoga on mood and anxiety found an increase in thalamic GABA levels, which are linked to decreased anxiety and an improved mood.

Today, many consider yoga as an effective way to regulate the functioning of the vagus nerve. To practitioners, the goal of yoga in relation to the vagus nerve is to become increasingly flexible in terms of the nervous system. Its main aim is to help people suffering from severe stress and trauma to become skilled in terms of switching between the parasympathetic and the sympathetic nervous system with less difficulty. Overall, yoga has been found to be good for improving the overall physical and mental health, although more research needs to be done on its impact on the vagal function.

Aerobics

Aerobics is another higher-intensity exercise, but some variants aren't as extensive or intensive as others. Zumba tends to be on the more intensive side, but there are different classes you can try. However, there are even different kinds of aerobic exercises, such as water aerobics, weight training, cycling, and even yoga.

All of these, when combined, are wonderful for vagus nerve stimulation and are great for the body. You'll be amazed and surprised at how helpful this can be for the body, and how you can use these to help improve your vagus nerve. They encourage you to breathe during these too, which promotes deep breathing and thereby, the vagus nerve stimulation.

Swim It Out!

Swimming is a great aerobic exercise too, and if you're not a fan of jogging or running, or weight training, swimming is good.

That's because it helps in many different ways. For starters, you're submerging your head, which stimulates the mammalian diving reflex, which includes your vagus nerve. It also pushes you to control your breathing as you move. You need to hold your breath, but also walk through the water, and it's a combination of both of those things which provides you with the correct vagus nerve stimulation.

It also will help improve your bodily movement. That's because you're moving about, and this encourages blood flow too. You'll notice that as you begin with this, it's hard to do, but over time, you'll get better with this. It's a beautiful form of cardio, and it's gorgeous for properly stimulating the vagus nerve.

Dancing

Dancing is an excellent form of self-expression for starters. Even if you're silly, it can help you feel much better about yourself. Dance is lovely because it enables you to improve your physical fitness, get the blood flow moving, and help you stay active and fun.

There are so many different kinds of dance classes these days too. You can do Zumba or other forms of dancing. Some people even like ballet dancing because it requires control, and this can stimulate the vagus nerve. They're fun to do, and they encourage you to move, control your breathing, and let you express yourself.

Even silly interpretive dancing helps. After all, if it can make you laugh, that naturally stimulates the vagus nerve, and that's a beautiful, fun way to do this.

Dancing is excellent, and it lets you feel good about yourself. Consider dancing the other time you want to express yourself correctly and feel good.

When it comes to stimulating the vagus nerve, these are all practice activities that boost the vagus nerve. Your vagus nerve is vital because it lets you relax the body and helps curb inflammation. But, while these exercises are great for stimulating this, it also helps with getting the body moving, which increases the vagal tone. It can also help offset obesity, diabetes, and other conditions related to weight.

Your vagus nerve does benefit from exercise, and here, we tackled why and how it happens, and the benefits of this.

High-Intensity Interval Sprinting

High-intensity interval sprinting stimulates the vagus nerve by waking up the heart and lungs. Doing these one to two times a week will provide the necessary stimulation to the nerve.

To do this exercise, run as fast as you possibly can for 30 seconds, and then walk for two minutes. This is one cycle. Repeat this cycle for just 10 minutes to get a full workout.

Cardio Machines

Treadmills or other walking machines at the gym are great if you don't have a good place to walk outdoors. Especially for those who live in cold climates, taking advantage of a treadmill at the gym or even investing in one for the home is a good way to keep you walking every day, indoors or out.

Jump Rope

Did you ever jump or skip rope as a child? Believe it or not, this childhood game is a great way to get your heart beating and your lungs expanding with fresh air. Find a simple child's jump rope and jump for two to five minutes a day to stimulate the vagus nerve. This can be done indoors (of course), but if you can, try to do it outside to get the extra benefits of fresh air and sun exposure.

Resistance Training

Otherwise known as weightlifting, this does more than just grow the muscles in your arms and legs. It also stimulates the cardiovascular system and speeds up your metabolism, which, in turn, stimulates the vagus nerve. For the vagus nerve stimulation, resistance training should be done one to four times a week. You don't have to go to the gym and bench-press 200 pounds to activate the vagus nerve. There are some very simple exercises you can do at home to get your heart pumping and your vagus nerve working.

Push-ups

Slow and controlled is the best way to do push-ups. Lower yourself down and hold for two seconds. Then push yourself up and hold for two seconds. Repeat this for 10 cycles.

Chest Press

Lay on your back on the floor. Take a dumbbell in each hand. The weight can be as light or as heavy as you wish, as long as the weight is even on both sides. Hold the weights in your fists, with your fingers facing straight up toward the ceiling. Lift the weights straight up toward the ceiling and hold there for a moment. Bend your elbows to bring the weights back down toward your body. Hold for a moment, and then lift again. Repeat this for 10 cycles.

Squats

There's no need to add extra weight; the squat itself is enough to stimulate the vagus nerve. To do a squat, spread your legs a little wider than hip-width apart. Bend your knees and lower yourself down almost to the floor. Hold for a moment, then straighten the knees until you are back to a standing position. Repeat this for 10 cycles.

Chewing Gum

The vagus nerve is connected to the muscles in your throat and face. It's responsible for the secretion of saliva in the mouth, and it regulates almost all of the digestive properties. Chewing gum may seem like a simple action, but it actually stimulates all of these reactions in the body. Chewing one stick of sugarless gum a day is a very easy way to stimulate the vagus nerve and allow it to do its healing work.

Vagus Nerve Morning Stimulation Routine

Morning routines are said to steady our moods and create a stronger tolerance towards pain. Then refine your routines as time goes by.

Mindfulness Meditation to Focus the Mind

First, find a comfortable posture to lie or sit in. The idea is to stay in this posture for a minute to determine if this would not cause you discomfort during your meditation and break your routine. If you are sitting on a chair, place your feet firmly on the ground. If you are sitting on a cushion, you can opt to sit in the full meditation pose of the lotus or half lotus. Alternatively, have your legs comfortably crossed in front of you. Your hands may gently rest on your knees or mid-thigh, whichever suits you. Lastly, eyes can be closed or open. If open, they should be cast downward as if in introspection. Morning meditation is dedicated to taking out time for ourselves before all the other things around us that are demanding our time and energy.

Focus on your breath. Inhale and exhale. Pay attention to how your chest rises and falls. A person's breath is consistent, always recurring in a similar fashion. Let your thoughts mull about. Trust that they will fade away with your breath and new ones will return with a breath.

Feel your body. As you continue to breathe, move your attention to the effect that the meditation has on your body. Let yourself feel the temperature of the room and the changes in light and sounds filtering in from the outside world.

Bring yourself back from the swirling emotions and thoughts. If the mind wanders to thoughts, center yourself to focus on the breath and nothing else. Inhale, exhale, and repeat. The concept of this morning meditation is to work on being present in the moment. Random thoughts might arise, such as *"We waste so much food. Why do we waste food? Is there perhaps something to do with the waste? What can I do better?"* Also, we might be confronted with more emotionally fueled thoughts, such as 'I love' or 'I hate.' The mind wanders. Regardless of which thoughts you experience, they keep on returning. The art is to realize the thought and see it pass.

Continue the mindfulness meditation for 15 minutes. When the time finally comes to wrap up, end the exercise slowly by opening your eyes and staying seated in the position for a further few minutes to acclimatize to the world around you.

This mindfulness meditation does not require you to be at home. This can be done even at work or in a quiet location outside. Find the time and dedicate that time to yourself!

Morning Pep Talk

Try reciting the following affirmations to increase your vagal tone. This practice will put you in a positive mood and enable you to face the day without any ill thoughts. Spend a minute or two on each affirmation.

- *"You have unlimited power!"*

- *"You are courageous."*

- *"You are enough. You will always be enough."*

- *"You have the grit to encourage positive change within your life."*

- *"You are of value and make notable contributions to the world and those around you."*

- *"You are a brave person who can and will attract success."*

- *"You are grateful and thankful for the life you have."*

- *"You are fearless and able to tackle any task or fear."*

- *"You can accept those who have different ideas or opinions."*

- *"You have all that you need to make this day wonderful."*

- *"You can love, and you will love."*

- *"You are living to your full potential."*

- *"You are surrounded by people who love you."*

- *"You are filled with great ideas."*

- *"Today, you shall cast aside old bad habits and grasp at new positive habits."*

Loving-Kindness Meditation

- Find a secluded spot for yourself with no interruptions from the outside world. Remember to switch off your phone and all electronic devices if you find yourself indoors. You do not want your meditation to be interrupted, as that would defeat the purpose and end goal.

- Finally, seat yourself comfortably. You can sit or lie down for this exercise. Find a position that will not require you to adjust the pose and interfere with your meditation later on.

- Close your eyes, take deep breaths, and take a moment to center yourself.

- Imagine yourself experiencing absolute peace and balance. Understand that you are loved and are perfect the way you are. With every inhale, imagine positive feelings to enter your body. With every exhale, imagine that tension and stress are leaving your body.

- Repeat the following sentences silently to yourself:

  o *"You can and will be happy."*

- o *"You can and will be safe."*

- o *"You are healthy, loving, and strong."*

- o *"You will receive and give kindness today."*

- Soak yourself in these affirmations and feelings of positivity.

- Focus on your breath and the affirmations.

- At your own time, move your focus to wishing peace, love, and joy onto those closest to you, such as family and close friends.

- Once you have focused your best intention upon yourself and loved ones, move your attention to wishing only good health and prosperity for those who also come into contact with you during your day.

- Gradually expand to wishing health, peace, and love unto all those in the world.

- When you feel that you have spent enough time on your meditation, you may open your eyes and gently bring yourself to awareness.

- It is suggested that you revisit the feelings that you had during your meditation throughout your day.

Tip: You can set yourself a gentle alarm to rouse you from your meditation if you only have a few minutes a day to commit to the practice. The above meditation is only a guideline to the practice, and you are welcome to change it to suit your needs.

Kundalini Morning Mantra

There is no need to get out of bed in the morning if you are going to practice this morning mantra. As mentioned, Kundalini yoga is a therapy that touches on every facet of your being, providing you the energy and motivation to embrace your day without stress. The mantra you can follow is 'sa, ta, na, ma.' It holds a very clear message and does not require any sudden movements or complex poses. The meaning of this mantra is as follows:

- **Sa**: Infinity

- **Ta**: Life

- **Na**: Death

- **Ma**: Rebirth

Let us begin:

Stretch and loosen your muscles when waking.

Sit upright in your bed, with your legs comfortably crossed.

Settle into your breathing.

Raise your arms out ahead of you, palms facing down, and think/whisper/say out loud, "Sa."

From this position, move your arms and hands upward, parallel to your ears, palms facing inward, and recite the word "Ta."

Lower your straightened arms alongside you, as if you need to touch the walls on your left-and right-hand side. Your arms, hands, and fingers should all be straight and aligned with your shoulders. Now say, "Na."

Lastly, bring your arms straight down alongside you and finish by saying, "Ma."

Repeat until you feel you are ready to leave your bed.

Here is an alternative Kundalini morning mantra:

- Stretch and loosen your muscles when waking.

- Sit upright in your bed, with your legs comfortably crossed.

- Settle into your breathing.

- Put your hands on your knees with palms facing up.

- Make the index finger and thumb touch each other and think/whisper/say out loud, "Sa."

- Make the middle finger and thumb touch each other and think/whisper/say out loud, "Ta."

- Make the ring finger and thumb touch each other and think/whisper/say out loud, "Na."

- Make the pinkie and thumb touch each other and think/whisper/say out loud, "Ma."

- The combination of movement, sound, and focus is a wonderful way to start your day!

Chapter 8: Measuring Vagal Tone with the Heart Rate Variability

Vagal Tone and Why It Matters

V agal tone is an important body parameter. This is because of the significance of the vagal nerve to the body. Essential body functions that are automated and isolated from conscious control are all moderated by the vagal nerve. For optimal healthy performance, the vagal nerve must be in a good condition. Vagal tone is used to determine the state of the vagal nerve. It tells us the present condition of the vagal nerve and helps us identify the effects that would be associated with such manifestation. From numerous researches, scientists have been able to come up with effective ways of distinguishing the common types of vagal tone the body experiences. The classification modes are the high vagal tone and the low vagal tone.

High Vagal Tone

The increase in the vagal tone of the body has been identified as a good phenomenon. Good in the sense that so many body functions are carried out optimally when the vagal tone is high. Since the vagal nerve is one of the most important cranial nerves and, in fact, the most complicated, its significance is too much to neglect.

Many people complain of difficulties having their blood regulated and distributed effectively around the body. This challenge is associated with a low vagal tone. When the vagal tone of an individual is relatively high, you can be rest assured that he/she would have better blood and sugar regulation. Blood regulation, which includes blood pressure, and heart rate, is essential for the body to remain in its state of equilibrium. The rate at which blood leaves the heart into the other areas of the body is what determines the ability of the heart to carry out its basic procedures.

With the emergence of better blood distribution, heart complications like strokes are avoided. Stroke is a medical condition arising from the inability of the blood to get to certain areas of the body. Stroke is not limited to any part of the body as any shortage of blood flow will eventually bring about this disease condition. High vagal tone is also accompanied with better digestion as enzymes that control the digestive processes are most readily released due to the communication between the stomach and the brain. Without the communication of this information with the brain on the type of food to be broken down, the brain cannot prescribe the appropriate enzyme to be produced. The inability of the body to engage in proper digestion only brings about complications and medical consequences. Another important aspect of having a high vagal tone is the ability of an individual to have a better mood and less anxious emotions. This, on its own, is a stress relief that helps the body in dealing with stress.

Low Vagal Tone

The decrease in the value of measured vagal time can be said to have its effects on various body operations. As much as this needs to be avoided, we must first understand its implications to the human body. Not many are aware of the dangers that are connected with having a low vagal tone. This is why they have paid little or/no attention to know what the state of their vagal tone is.

One of the dangers of having a low vagal tone is cardiovascular conditions. These conditions are associated with the heart. The heart is a very delicate organ and must be treated with care. The neurons and control mechanisms that automate activities must ensure that it functions at the optimum capacity. Heart conditions may result from the inability of the blood being pumped to be circulated around the entire body, creating room for the decay of some organs or death of cells.

Another implication of a low vagal tone is depression. This has been at the peak of emotional disorders and conditions faced by today's world. You have lots of young and aged people going into depression of varying degrees. Some have attributed it to some spiritual or mystic event. They are still ignorant that feelings and emotions are impulses that are sent from the brain. The inability of the vagus nerve to pick up these signals or picking it up at reduced speed can bring an individual into a state of depression. Depression can be triggered by a lot of factors, both psychological and physiological. When depressive moods begin to set in, it is the duty of the vagus nerve to release anti-depressing hormones to counteract the reaction.

Chronic fatigue syndrome is another associated phenomenon with a low vagal tone. This arises from the continued tiredness experienced by the body, even when it shouldn't. This will make an individual feel weak most of the time and induce lesser productivity. People with this kind of condition have difficulties carrying out predefined tasks and objectives. They are not in control of when the feeling of tiredness would set in. They are only accustomed to the feelings when it fully manifests.

People with a low vagal tone should also be prepared to face serious inflammatory conditions. These arise from the inability of the immune system to secret anti-inflammatory antigens to defend the body. This especially can bring about different types of health conditions like bowel diseases, arthritis and so many others. The brain's inability to send information to the immune system to begin deployment of antibodies will further complicate the situation on the ground. It is advisable to perform regular checkups to avoid your vagal tone from depreciating that much.

Measuring Your Vagal Tone

The measurement of the vagal tone comes with a scientific method. A common method being applied today is the heart rate count during breathing. When you take in air and breathe out the waste, there is always a rhythm and rate at which your heart produces. This heart rate speeds up a little when air is being taken into the body. It is slower when exhalation takes place. The difference in the heart rate between inhalation and exhalation gives an idea of how low or high the vagal tone is.

What is the Heart Rate Variability?

The heart rate variability looks at the intervals between consecutive heartbeats in milliseconds, and determines the variation. Our heart does not tick evenly throughout the day. It actually varies tremendously. HRV is not the same as counting your heartbeat per minute. We are not acutely aware of this change within milliseconds, and specialized tools are needed to accurately assess HRV. One of the key points to take away from here is that the time between each consecutive heartbeat is different from beat to beat. It is never completely uniform. An example of when variation occurs is when we inhale and exhale. When we inhale, our HRV decreases, meaning the distance and time between beats is shorter. When we exhale, our HRV increases, meaning the distance between beats becomes longer. HRV also increases with exercises and other strenuous activities.

The main thing to understand is that the higher a person's HRV, the healthier their autonomic nervous system is. This is because a higher HRV indicates more resiliency and flexibility in the function of the heart. The heart is able to adjust more quickly when it has a higher HRV in general, and this allows it to respond to the needs of the body. A lower HRV has been shown to correlate with higher levels of illness and morbidity. Try assessing your HRV by counting your pulse and assessing the difference in time between beats from when you inhale and exhale. This will showcase your HRV.

The reason this is important is that many of the exercises we will mention work by increasing our heart rate variability. Increasing our vagal tone immensely improves upon this factor and improves our heart function. Heart rate is directly impacted by the autonomic nervous system, so increasing its ability to control the heart rate through a properly functioning vagus nerve is critical.

We discussed various ways to test the vagus nerve function in this chapter. We also mentioned the study conducted by Dr. Stephen Porges. An objective way you can test your vagus nerve is by assessing your heart rate variability. One way is by counting the variation in beats during different portions of breathing. Also, you may check your HRV when you exercise to see how much it increases from your resting state. HRV is a good self-assessment in determining the health of the vagus nerve.

Heart rate variability is simply the measure of the difference between two successive heartbeats. The optimum functioning of the heartbeat at times when the body is resting is so that the body cells don't die due to shortages in blood and oxygen. The red blood cells are what carry the oxygen to the distinct parts of the body. The regulation of the heart rate isn't controlled by your conscious desire to do so. It is already built into your brain system to exert a great amount of influence on the heart rate. Have you imagined why your heartbeat tends to go up faster when you have increased brain activity? It is because your brain activity has been set to have a direct effect on the heart and rate of blood flow.

The same way breathing and digestion are being controlled and automated, is the same way the heart functions are regulated. The autonomic nervous system can also be subdivided into the sympathetic and parasympathetic, respectively. The parasympathetic components can be tagged as the flight and response mechanism. This part of the nervous system is what gives you the urge to take action when an activity threatens the state of safety.

The brain works like a computer, carrying out diverse kinds of information processing. Through the help of the autonomic nervous system, signals are being sent to various parts of the body to trigger the implementation of various activities. This response is not limited to a bad day at the office, or when a piece of exciting news is mentioned, with our bodies having different ways of dealing with shock or when excited. This is accompanied by a spike or reduction in the rate at which blood is being pumped. The balance of this response and trigger can be taken off with a balance on things like a healthy diet, relationships, and exercise.

Why Check Heart Rate Variability?

Heart rate variability is a very good tool for the identification of imbalances that are associated with the autonomic nervous system. The ability of an individual to switch moods from one to another is a good reason for this analysis. The heartbeat when a person is in his/her flight mode is always high. This can be used to test for the health of the vagal tone. The speed with which an individual can switch modes is attributed to the health of his autonomous nervous system. Research over the years has brought to light the relationship between the low heart rate variability and the increasing depression cases. This can be a source of deaths emanating from heart diseases.

Higher heart rate variability will help the individual maintain better cardiovascular conditions and create a defense system against the effect of stress. It can also be used to determine the kind of lifestyle being lived and can help with improving one's way of living. HRV has also been said to have a transforming effect on the physical attributes of the individual, which might include sleep, mindfulness, meditation and the rest. You can now be sure that your nervous system is still on track and free from the influence of emotions, thoughts and feelings.

Measuring Nervous Function with Heart Rate Variability (HRV)

We saw earlier what the HRV is all about. This time, we are going to take a closer look at the concept and how it can be used to measure the functioning of the vagus nerve.

An important thing to note is that the HRV is a non-invasive method of measuring the Autonomic Nervous System (ANS).

Typically, the heart rate of a person is used to understand a lot of factors. The high heart rate typically means that the person has a high blood pressure or might be suffering from anxiety. But when you use HRV, you get a more accurate understanding of how the autonomic nervous system is functioning. Here are some of the things that you can understand using HRV:

- How well you recover from stress

- The body's resilience and ways to improve it

- Optimizing physical training and recovery of the heart from anxiety and other situations

- Help with sleep and nutrition

- Improve mental health; mood, depression, anxiety

- Improve mental performance and cognition

- Identify the risk of diseases

- Measure the inflammation rate in our bodies

- Bring balance to the nervous system

- Discover any changes to the health and wellbeing of the person

Think about it. We can get a whole lot more data about the nervous system when we make use of the HRV. It is like opening a big encyclopedia and finding out the information that we require.

Interpreting the Heart Rate Variability Results

One thing to note is that the heart rate is one essential metric value whose determination lies not just on the speed of blood being pumped, but on the timely variations that spike with each heartbeat. It has been already seen that individuals with a higher HRV (heart rate variability) result come out having better health when compared to individuals with a lower HRV. This is so because their hearts are more active, thus increasing the ability of the heart to take more desired volumes of blood to different parts of the body when needed. This activity can also be seen as a means of disease prevention. It is being said that as blood flows through the blood veins, it takes along with it the contamination that would have constituted ill health.

This is true for many reasons; one of them being that persons with increased blood activity either through daily exercise or muscle activity have reduced risks of falling ill. This can be well seen in athletics and sportsmen. For the human body to remain in healthy conditions, blood flow accompanied by a good heart rate should be maintained. A low heart rate variability result gives rise to the formation of many killer disease conditions. Having a low HRV doesn't necessarily mean that the disease condition has been formed yet, but with time the strength of the body in fighting against most of these infections would be reduced.

The HRV data isn't just significant to heart conditions alone. It can also be used to reduce emotional, mental and behavioral patterns. Studies have shown that the emotional state of an individual has a direct relationship in the results of an HRV test. For example, a man who just came back from his office, where he just received a promotion would have a happy and excited emotional state. This state of excitement would give birth to a high HRV value. This can be characterized by reduced cause for worry, less formation of disease conditions and so on.

Medical experts have informed us that the more a man stays happy, the healthier he tends to become. This emanated from the series of experiments carried out on various calibers of individuals. The results came out with those having better minds and happy emotions living above the expected medical threshold. Worries, anxiety and fear are all sources of health drains. The time spent thinking and worrying about the state of things could be invested in making the most of life. You can even discover that your most productive moments come at times when you are better relaxed, happy and in no sad emotional state. Thoughts and ideas seem to flow perfectly, reducing the risks of brain fatigue.

Another revelation by research has been the dependence of the HRV values on other factors like self-control. Self-control arises from the ability of the individual to be self-aware of himself. His control over his entire body comes from his ability to take control of his mental activities. Putting to check the thoughts he allows into his mind, exercises the control of his entire body and mental activity.

The stress that comes with rigorous brain activity can be filtered to a large extent. Self-control is a deliberate act, where you try to possess conscious power over your mind and life. Most motivational speakers challenge you to take control of your life by charting the way forward through ideas and innovations. This cannot be possible when you have lots of things to worry about. Editing these time and energy wasters will give you the required energy to break past your limitations.

Stress management, as advised by many, is better achieved when individuals pay attention to managing all that comes to reduce or abnormally increase the heart rate. Though heart rate should be moderately high, it doesn't permit excessively high heart rates. The higher the heart rate is above normal, the more dreadful it becomes. Many with good social skills have been traced back to healthy emotional and heart conditions. The happiness an individual exhibits can be transmitted to all those around, thus helping him connect better with people. You can now see that the applications of the heart rate variability give beyond just medical examination and benefits, but also into the social world. Imagine the fact that a good HRV value could just be the reason why you get the next promotion at the office due to an increased productivity and efficient service delivery. It could also be the reason why your relationship issues with those around you gets resolved.

The arousal for the tendencies for physiological stress can be well monitored through HRV tests. This can predict and show you the occurrences of a low heart rate variability value. The awareness of this result will guide you in making healthier choices that will eliminate the challenges that come with such. Investigation can be carried out through varying methods.

These methods can include the ECG (Electrocardiogram) devices.

When we try to analyze the little differences present in the interval between heartbeats, we attempt to trace the signals that create the heart heat to the sources where they are coming from. This could be the SNS (Sympathetic Nervous System) or PNS (Parasympathetic Nervous System). The PNS and SNS are collectively responsible for making and establishing the heartbeats knowing that the body system that is active will give the necessary information on the level of stress received by the body, and how well it copes under pressure.

There are two known methods for analyzing the heart rate variability. They are the time domain and the frequency domain analysis. In both methods, the interval between the heartbeats is measured. This could also be called the RR-intervals.

Time-Domain Analysis

The time-domain analysis tells how the HRV tends to change as time progresses. It can also be used to estimate the sympathetic and parasympathetic activity. Among the many domain characters used are RR, SDNN, TINN, *etc.*

When grouping, intervals are placed in bands according to their length. An example would be placing them in bands like 700-800, 500-600, and 800-900 ms. The intervals are then categorized to see how many of them would fall into the bands allocated.

Frequency-Domain Analysis

To be able to identify the process that the body is undergoing, we would carry out a frequency domain analysis. This will tell us if the body is currently undergoing recovery or stress. Knowledge of what process is being carried out will help us know how to manage the conditions and channel the energy towards the most productive outcome. For recovery processes, the body is trying to regain its lost energy. The heart-pumping rate at this point is quite faster than normal, especially as we apply procedures to increase the heart rate significantly. For stress processes, the body needs to reduce the heart rate significantly.

In the extraction of these parameters, each length of the interval is changed into waves so that the frequencies can be measured. The waves are separated into low and high frequencies and very low-frequency bands.

The analysis of the parameters mentioned will give doctors and health coaches the knowledge of the body's coping mechanism with pressure, the effect of changes like stress, relocation to zero gravity surroundings, and the increase in workout loads. The unfortunate thing is that the interpretation of high rate variability data isn't a universal experiment where the values could be generalized for all cases. You can have a varying number of factors that could be at play, which would cause fluctuations of results. An example of such a fracture would be the time at which the individual's nervous system responds more to the stress signals, post HRV measurement results, *etc.* What could be an indication of high stress for one, might to our surprise, be in a normal range for someone else. This has made us confine HRV to remote fields like space, medicine and sports. This can afford much time and resources for tests to be carried out in one person.

Welltory Provides Personalized HRV Interpretations without Labs Tests

A new technology has been developed, which gives more specific interpretation of the HRV. This method utilizes data by automating the processes previously carried out manually. The main advantage over the other methods is the vast database comprising over two million HRV measurements, already enriched with health and lifestyle data. You can imagine having two million data points to work with; and you can be sure of a better accuracy.

With this technology, people are separated into four nervous type systems aided through the big data tech. The result of these categories is tested against five thousand already done clinical assessments, which have been completed by the previous users. This gave birth to the world's first self-learning HRV algorithm, capable of adapting to various nervous systems of different individuals. The algorithm developed also accounts for factors like age, gender, the time of the day and even results from past measurements.

To enable an application that is easy to use and well simplified, the standard list of parameters with health scores are replaced with others most easily understood. The scores are accompanied by data driven recommendations, which help people feel better every day. The recommendations can help the individual live a healthier life free of HRV complications.

Increasing Your Vagal Tone

There are various methods that can be applied to improving the vagal tone. Since there is an increased awareness of the advantages and benefits of having a good vagal tone, the question about how to go about this has risen in different folds. It is one thing to know the importance of something and another to know how to go about it. The methods listed below have a proven result rate. By carefully applying the methods suggested here, you can be rest assured that you would generate higher vagal tones. These methods aren't so sophisticated or scientifically driven so that even the most ignorant individuals can achieve the same results. To be able to improve your vagal tone, you need to center your efforts on the parts that have a direct relationship with the vagal nerve.

The human body is, by default, trained to breathe from the lungs. This breathing pattern doesn't allow for a more calm and relaxed result. You would notice that most times, when you attempt breathing heavily, your body movement is centered around your chest area. This signifies that your breathing systems are centered around the lungs and not from the diaphragm. You would need to readjust your system to get used to breathing from your diaphragm. This enables you to maintain slow and rhythmic breathing patterns. This, in turn, helps your vagal nerves become more relaxed and at an appropriate level. This has a direct impact on your heart rate as your heart beats become more organized in the most suitable manner. Better blood diffusion into the different body organs and systems can only be possible when breathing is carried out from the diaphragm. How to perform slow breathing is discussed in subsequent pages of this book.

Humming

Another relaxing technique is the application of humming. Hums come from audible sounds that are made by vibrations on your vocal cords. The biological arrangement of the vocal cords is in such a way that the vagus nerves are connected to them. The importance of this is the fact that vibrations along the vocal cords would automatically trigger the vagus nerve to perform better. As simple as this method seems, it is a very efficient way to trigger the vagus nerve, it is being referred mostly as a mechanical method. While humming, the individual might choose to make use of alphabets or words. Constant practice of this method will ensure an increased vagal tonal result. This is why singers and vocal artists have higher chances of possessing better vocal tones; the frequent vibration of their vocal cords enables such responses. You don't necessarily need to be a musician to achieve the desired result. All you need to do is make sure you consistently keep to the humming routine. Most people prefer to use sentences while humming. It should be noted that there are no specific benchmarks on what to hum.

Speaking

Another method that could be used to stimulate the vagus nerve is speaking. Like humming, it has to do with sounds that are generated through the vibration of the vocal cords. Speaking at minimized levels helps keep the vibrations sufficient enough to evoke a response on the vagal nerve. This type of speaking doesn't mean that your voice must be pitched at a certain level. The theory of sound production in the mouth is brought about by the vibration of waves. To eliminate the adverse effect of this method, individuals are advised to mind the number of hours spent on talking. As much as the procedure can bring tangible results, you should also know that talking is energy-draining/consuming. You should then be mindful of the degree to which you engage this method to avoid adding more stress to the body.

Mediation

This is a very effective tool being deployed in the vagal tone increment. To carry this out, the individual is advised to focus his/her thoughts on good memories of himself, acts of love and kindness, and so on. By constantly doing so, the vagus nerve devices are stimulated more to function better. A study carried out in 2010 shows that positive emotions have a direct effect on the social engagement of a person, which in turn affects the vagus nerve. Sadness is an emotional condition associated with a low vagal tone. Since the motive behind all of this is to increase the vagal tone, anything capable of helping the mind get into an excited state is welcomed. At this point, many neurons are more fired up and ready to transmit signals. The nervous system is said to be at the peak of its performance at this period. You must guard against worries, events and situations that come to induce sadness and sorrow if you must see that your vagal tone doesn't depreciate.

Balancing the Gut Microbiome

Micro biomes are small bacteria that can be found in the gut tracks. The presence of these microorganisms helps to improve the tone of the vagal nerve.

These simple procedures have an implication on the general health of the individual. They have far-reaching positive effects; they also include the prevention of inflammations. Inflammations could be very expensive to treat and manage, which makes prevention a better option. Since the application of these exercises ensures, to a large extent, the prevention of inflammation, they should be encouraged more for every person. Other conditions that are also avoided include digestive upsets arising from the inability of the vagus nerve to carry out hormonal indicators for the production of necessary digestive enzymes. You can also prevent high blood pressure-related diseases. Most of these diseases come from the inability of the heart to regulate itself.

Vagal tone exercises are also a recommended preventive action for depression cases. Meditation, which is very helpful to human health, contributes its role to the elevation of the self-esteem of the individual, and brings positive thoughts to the mind of the individual. Depression emanates from the lack of belief and trust in one's own self. This would progress to suicidal and low living standards. A good vagal tone can help prevent all these possibilities. Studies have shown that individuals who have a low vagal tone end up having more signs of depression than others.

Conclusion

T his book is not the beginning or the end of the discussion on the vagus nerve. It was intended to introduce you to the vagus nerve, it is still just a starting point, but it is easy to read and understand. Maybe after you have read this book and you have tried the exercises; it will spark more interest in you. The vagus nerve is not a new discovery, most people are just not aware about it.

The vagus nerve is connected to many parts of our bodies, and as such, it has been found that we can activate it naturally using these parts of our bodies to stimulate it. An active vagus nerve means that our bodies can achieve a state of equilibrium between the parasympathetic and sympathetic nervous systems. When either system is not balanced out by the actions of the other, we tend to develop physical and psychological disorders that impact our quality of life.

Living with depression and anxiety can seem like a jail sentence of sorts except you're a prisoner of your own mind. They are debilitating states of mind to live with and it will often seem that there are no options or ways out of the mess you find yourself in. As you've seen throughout this book, this does not have to be the case.

The fact is that your body already has everything it needs to heal you and fight back against all that ails it. It's merely a question of aligning yourself with the things that prompt your body to spring into action. The link between your mind and your actions goes both ways.

Set long-term goals for yourself, at least a year out, and live every day as you need to. Focus on carrying out the treatment methods I've listed in this book and do what you need to do to feel good. I guarantee you that by the end of the time frame you have in mind to achieve your goal, you'll be a changed person.

Learning this information will help your brain convince itself that the vagus nerve holds the power to heal you and that all of the treatment options are medically sound.

Exercising control over the nervous system seems to be a big deal for many people. This has led to frustration when faced with challenges like stress, anxiety, depression and so on, and has unfortunately for many, led to their untimely death.

To be able to stimulate the vagus nerve to function properly, you need to take a look at its structure, anatomy and its general functions. This will arm you with adequate knowledge on how best to get this nerve to work optimally.

With the points discussed in this book, you now better understand the different health conditions that can result when the vagus nerve is damaged and why you should be careful of the food and substances allowed into your body. Above all, with the methods of stimulation discussed in the pages of this book, you are now equipped to taking charge of your health and wellbeing for good by practicing any of the methods that are comfortable for you, depending on your current health situation.

Finally, I urge you to take personal responsibility for your health by making the tips shared in this book become a part of your daily life routine.

Harnessing the hidden power of the vagus nerve is not a contradiction of medical science, neither is it declaring war on therapy, but like every genuine and powerful healing principle, it is to be applied along with modern medicine. Pick up the slack when medicine wavers or take a generalized and counterproductive approach to some cases.

All that you need to do is take action and remember that you are worth it. Always. I wish you the best of luck and all the peace in the world!

Printed in Great Britain
by Amazon